SYSTEMA PARTNER TRAINING

Robert Poyton

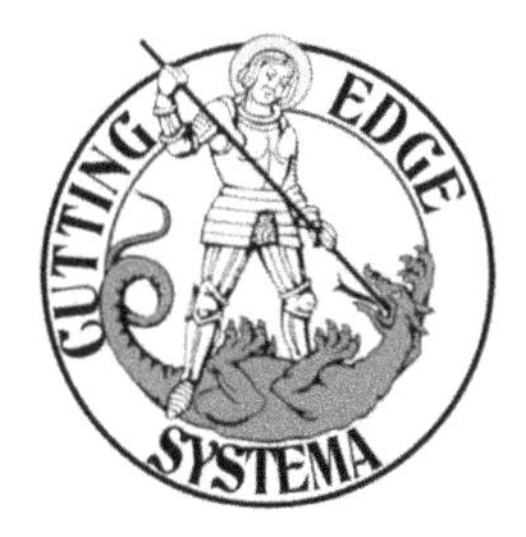

Published by Cutting Edge

ISBN: 978-0-9956454-8-6

DEDICATIONS

With respect and gratitude to Mikhail Ryabko,
and Vladimir and Valerie Vasiliev
for their generosity and guidance.

Thanks to all my regular friends and students
and everyone else who helped
in the production of this book.

ABOUT THE AUTHOR

Robert was born in the early 1960's in East London.
He trained in Judo and boxing as a child and at age
18 began training in Yang Family Taijiquan.

For many years he studied the Chinese Internal Arts in depth.
In the 1990's he set up his own school and began cross
training in several styles.

Robert trained with Vladimir Vasiliev on his first visit to the UK
in 2001 and has trained at Vladimir's Toronto school
several times. He has also travelled to Moscow for intensive
training with Mikhail Ryabko and his senior instructors.
In addition he has arranged numerous UK seminars for
Mikhail, Vladimir and other leading instructors.

Robert now trains solely in Systema and was one
of the first registered UK instructors. He runs regular classes
and workshops in the UK and teaches seminars throughout
the UK and Europe.

He has been featured in numerous martial arts books
and magazines as well as producing his own
magazines and training films.

Outside of training Robert is a professional musician
and currently lives in rural Bedfordshire with his wife
and several chickens.

CONTENTS

CHAPTER ONE
INTRODUCTION

"It takes two flints to make a fire."

— Louisa May Alcott.

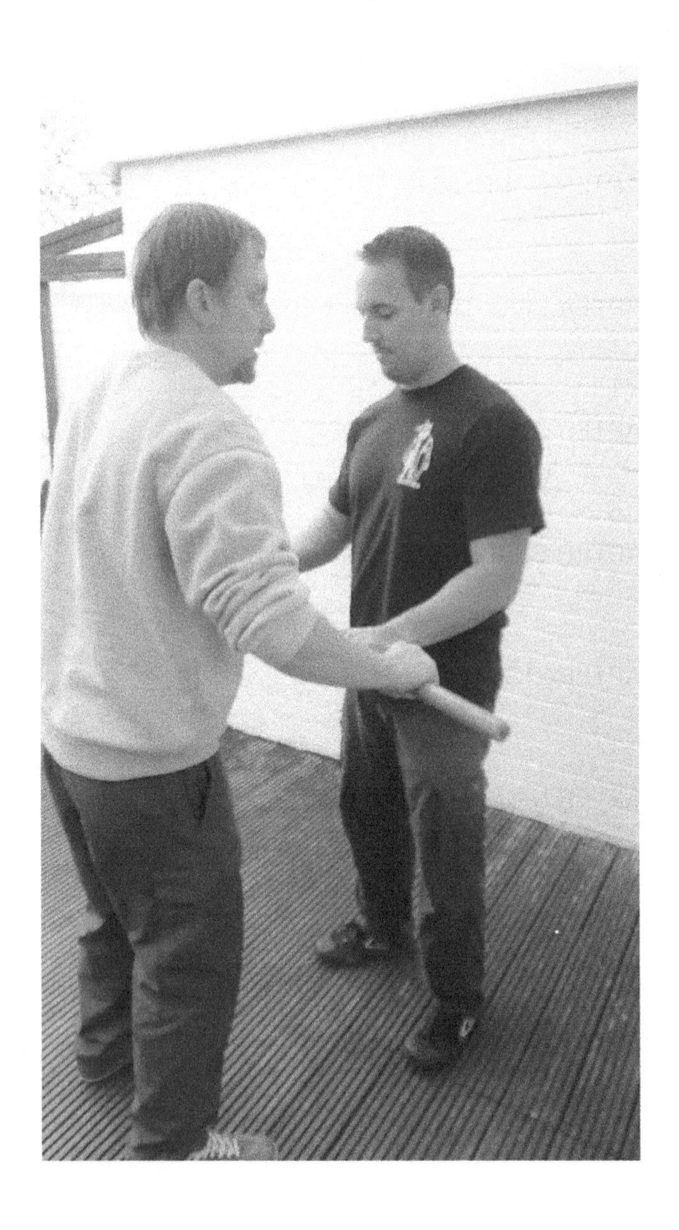

PARTNER TRAINING

In our last book we looked at ideas for training alone from a Systema perspective. This, of course, is useful for those times when we have no training partner available but still wish to develop the attributes required for our Systema work. As we mentioned in that book, we can exercise "alone in a group" and this is a feature of most Systema classes, for reasons we discussed before.

But are there methods of exercise we can do with a partner or in a group? The answer is yes! So in this book we have set out some ideas for training in pairs, threes, fours, or even larger groups.

I would like to stress at the start that we have tried to keep to exercises in this book (mostly working on strength and structure) rather than drills or direct application work. See Vladimir Vasiliev's *Strikes*, Matt Hill's *Systema Combat Drills* or our own *Ten Points of Sparring* for some ideas on those. But it is a thin line between practice and application in Systema and we know that attributes developed during exercise form an important part of our applied work. Systema exercises help provide the structure, movement, fear control and so on that are so vital to "real life" work.

So, we of course get the same benefits from partner exercises as from solo exercise but are there other benefits too? I believe so. Working with a partner helps develop our sensitivity, whether it be touch, sight, awareness of breathing and so on. It helps develop the feel of contact with another body or bodies, sometimes in a challenging way.

We can gain a sense of how to support or help another person, in a physical and psychological sense - but be aware that does not mean always being "pleasant" to your partner!

Some work calls for us to help our partner by putting them under some kind of pressure, which can sometimes prove almost as challenging as being on the receiving end. But it is through discomfort that we develop and grow.

Working with others in this way is gives us a strong sense of teamwork, particularly in exercises that call for group cooperation. There are important life lessons to be learned here, for none of us is an island.

Naturally, all the same requirements from solo training are present in our partner work. Breathing, posture, awareness of tension, smooth movement. We will cover these again here in case you have not read the Solo Training. If you have read that book you can skip the next section.

One addition from solo training is sensitivity to our partner's abilities and needs and the requirement, always, for safe training practices. Here are some issues to bear in mind:

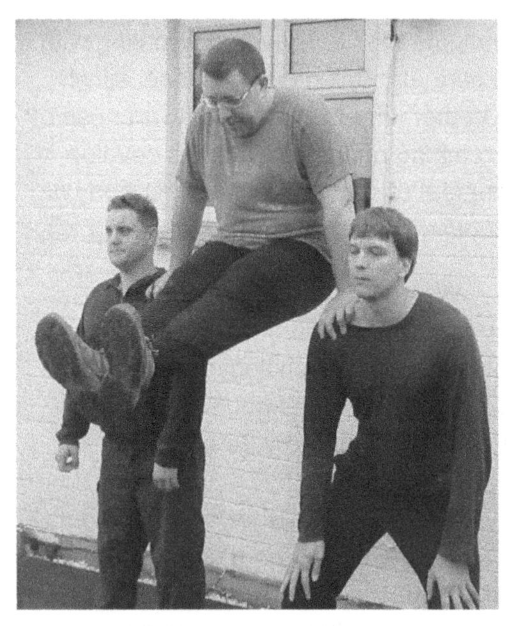

Never move your partner quickly or jerkily under tension.

Always apply just as much force or pressure as is required, not too much and not too little.

Constantly monitor each other for signs of distress or extreme discomfort.

Never move limbs outside of their natural range of motion.

Be aware of any injuries or problems you or your partner may have.

For more challenging or extreme work it is useful to have a prearranged "safe word". The instant the safe word is spoken, the exercise stops, without delay and without judgement!

Be aware of the purpose of the exercise and how best to help your partner achieve their goals.

Don't be lazy, embrace challenge and change. Be creative!

Always employ the correct breathing method - check out the material from Systema HQ for more guidelines and information

BASICS

There are certain principles that are fundamental requirements of Systema training and should be present in all activities. Whether engaging in solo or group training, we should always be mindful of these requirements.

THE FOUR PILLARS

Systema is often said to be built on four major principles - the Four Pillars. They are relaxation, form, movement and breathing. The practitioner should understand the role of each in any type of exercise or drill. We will briefly look at the first three principles in turn, then take a more in-depth look at breathing, as it is the most important of all.

Although we often separate them for ease of learning, we should remember that in reality there is constant inter-action between all of these principles. We should also bear in mind that there is a psychological as well as physical aspect to each principle too.

RELAXATION

In our activities we are looking to accomplish any given task with just the required amount of tension. If we look at fitness training in general it is not uncommon to see people doing fast squats with red faces and hunched up shoulders. People get the pulse elevated and so feel they are achieving something. Unfortunately all they are often doing is increasing the tension within the body with a corresponding risk to health.

For the most part we are seeking to perform any exercise or movement with the minimal amount of tension. For a push-up this means relaxing the shoulders, holding the body straight and keeping just enough tension in the hands and wrists to maintain the structure - think of the body as a bridge, it has to be strong in the right places, but if the whole structure is tense and immovable it will fail under load.

Some exercises call for us to tense muscles - either specific muscles or the whole body. The purpose of these exercises is usually to help us release accumulated tension, or in order to help strengthen a particular part of the body.

As we will see later, Systema stretching is built heavily on the idea of releasing tension rather than "stretching the muscle". We try and avoid moving under tension - or at least moving fast. Slow movement under tension can be useful for some things, but should always be done with care.

Try to get in the habit during the day of regularly "checking yourself" for

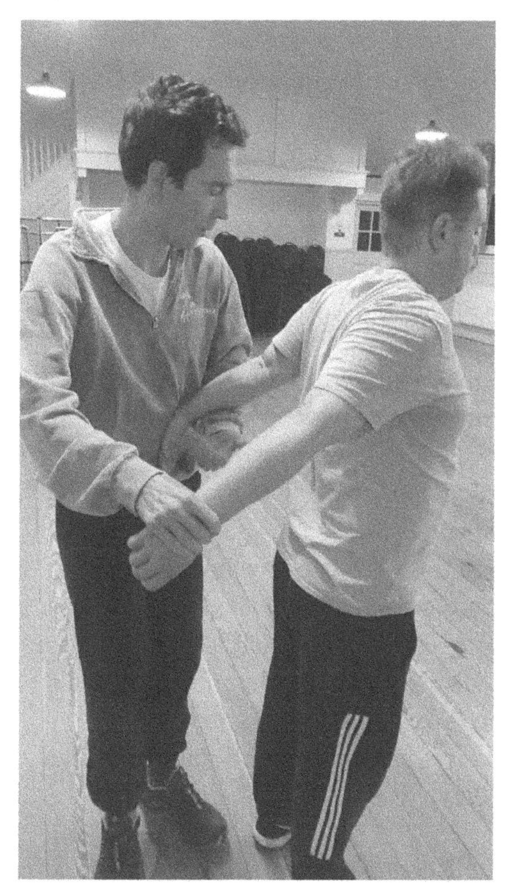

unwanted stress. Over time you will get a feeling for controlling your tension and how to get rid of any excess. This in itself is one of the greatest benefits of Systema training, as stress is a leading cause of numerous modern lifestyle ailments.

FORM

By form we mean good posture and practical knowledge of your body on a bio-mechanical level. As unwanted tension is released, you will find ways of using or organising your body structure with greater efficiency.

To return to our push-up example, you will find that with correct form you are able to "rest on the bones" rather than use tense muscles to support your body weight. Exactly the same principle applies to standing or sitting.

Achieving this in static posture is one thing, doing so in solo movement is another. Adding in pressure from outside in form of a partner or equipment adds in another level of challenge.

If you want to get a feel for good basic posture, simply stand upright and relax the body, without slouching. Imagine you are holding a stick across your shoulders (or actually use a stick). Your shoulders and hips should be level, it is surprising how many people carry one side higher than the other.

Check in a mirror or have someone correct you. Your head should not lean or jut forward. To get this feeling, place your hand on the crown of your head, grab some hair (if you have some!) and pull lightly upwards. You should feel the neck stretch slightly and the chin tuck in a little. This is the optimum position for the head. The spine too should be straight, with no lean or kinks. Think of the spine as an antenna, with the head atop. The better its shape, the more information it can take in and relay.

There are many resources available to learn about bio-mechanics and also many new developments going on in sports science. It is good to get a sound scientific understanding of how the body operates - as well , of course, as corresponding information on psychology and the like. However intellectual understanding is always a support to physical work and can never replace "body knowledge".

MOVEMENT

With relaxation and good posture comes free movement. Through correct exercise we can explore our range of motion, develop strength in different vectors, improve how we walk, run, climb and so on. I feel that freedom of body movement also brings with it a sense of liberation. It is hard to be "uptight" when the body is free and relaxed.

This takes us back to a time when we were children - watch how young kids move, often with very little tension and no preconceived notions or mental blockages.

The notion of "playfulness" is an important and powerful aspect of Systema training. Even the most challenging exercises should be approached with a focused but playful mindset rather than the "no pain no gain", suffering mindset. Pain is inevitable, suffering is optional!

BREATHING

No type of Systema training should be undertaken without at least a basic understanding of breathing.

We advise that you consult the many resources available from Systema HQ that go into greater detail, but here are some of basic methods to use when training.

Unless otherwise directed, the procedure is to inhale through the nose and exhale through the mouth. People typically exhale upon exertion, which is fine, but is is also good to get used to inhaling on exertion too.

Breathing should be comfortable, not over filling or completely emptying, unless otherwise directed. Learn to breathe smoothly and to the requirements of the situation.

When you first start out it is advisable to practice breathing in a safe and comfortable position. If you have any blood pressure or other health issues, always check with your healthcare professional prior to training.

DEPTH OF BREATHING

There are three main "depths" of breathing. The first is shallow or *burst breathing*. Think of a dog panting, the breath comes in the nose and straight out of the mouth. This is most often used as a recovery breath, or in stressful situations. So if your system is stressed you can use burst breathing to regain control and return to a state of equilibrium

The second is our normal, everyday chest breathing. The ribcage expands and contracts with each inhale and exhale. This may still be fairly shallow, or can be practiced more deeply. The main point to watch is that there is no unnecessary tension, particularly in the shoulders.

The third is abdominal breathing. This is where the diaphragm is fully used in order to draw and expel the breath. This can be "normal", where the diaphragm pushes out on the inhale, in on the exhale, or "reverse

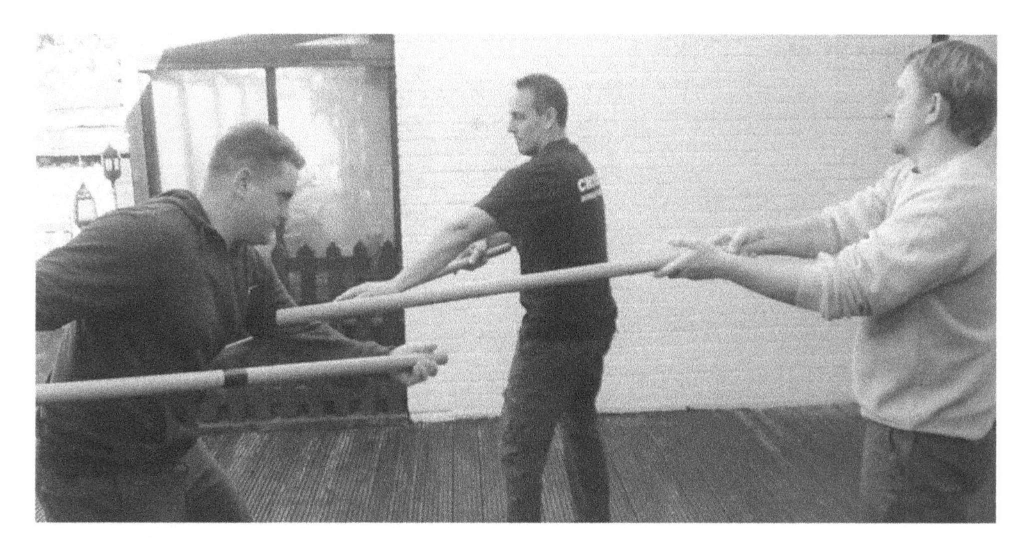

breathing" where the diaphragm pulls in and up on the inhale and expands out on the exhale.

We recommend you begin with chest breathing, then burst breathing for recovery. Deeper breathing is best trained under the supervision of a good Instructor. Here are some simple solo exercises to get you started.

Remember, check out the material from Systema HQ for more in-depth work. If at any time you feel dizzy, then come out of the exercise immediately and sit quietly to recover.

NORMAL BREATHING WITH TENSE / RELAX

Find a comfortable position, standing, sitting or prone. Inhale nose, exhale mouth for a while, slowing the breathing.

Then on the inhale, tense a body part. Just the one section, the rest of the body stays relaxed. Repeat two or three times. On the exhale, relax the body part. A typical sequence might be – legs, stomach, chest, back, shoulders, arms, head.

To finish, tense and relax the whole body three times on the inhale/exhale

WAVE BREATHING

On the inhale, tense the whole body, starting with the feet up to the crown of the head. The wave of tension matches the speed of the breathing. On the exhale, relax from the crown of the head to the feet. Do this three times then reverse the direction.

BREATH HOLDS AND RECOVERY

Inhale and hold for as long as you can. Do not overfill the lungs, work to about 80% capacity. Try and feel where the tension begins in your body. Work to move it or dissolve it. When you release, use burst breathing to recover. Repeat on an exhale/hold

PYRAMID BREATHING

Walk or jog – one step inhale, one step exhale. Gradually increase – 2, 3, 4 etc up to 10. Each time the breath should stretch over the amount of

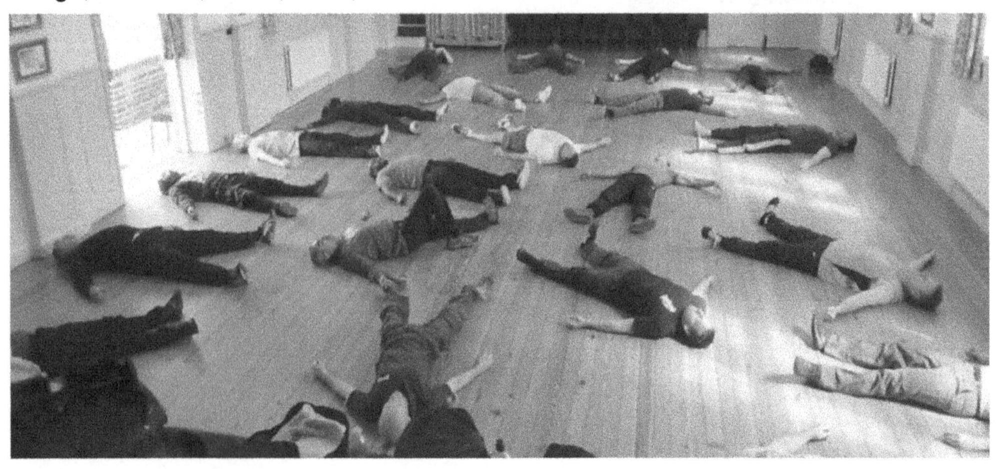

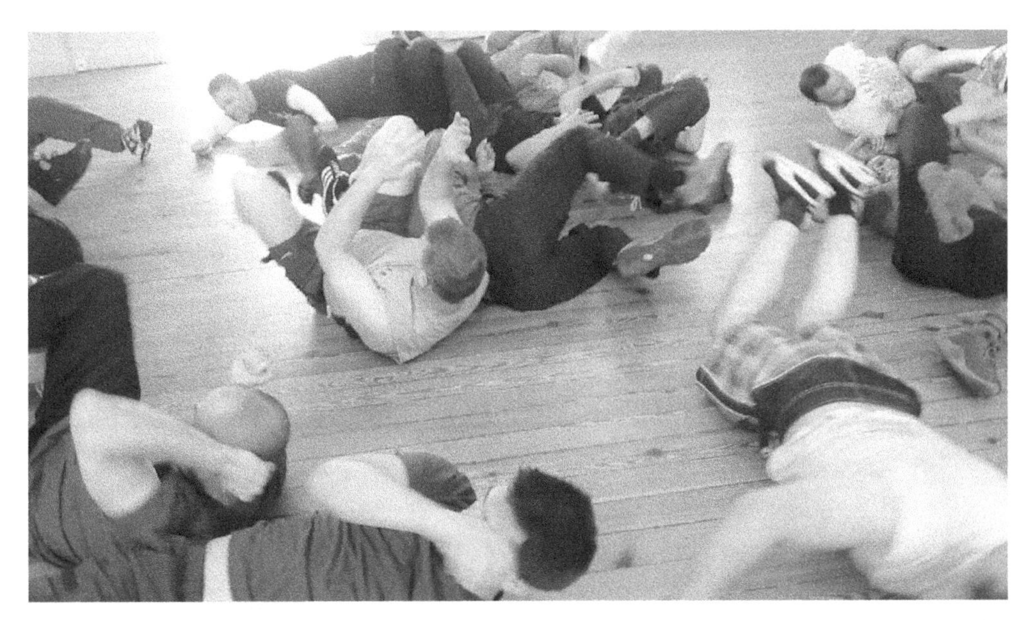

steps. From 10 work back down to 1 again. Take your time and work only up to your limit. Over time, push the limit

SQUARE BREATHING

This follows the same procedure as above, but you add in a breath hold. So inhale 2, hold 2, exhale 2, hold 2 and so on. You can increase the breath hold along with the step, or keep it at a constant number.

These are some basic patterns which we can be added into the various exercises described later. If no particular breathing pattern is described, then the default is to exhale on the exertion or the stretch. Unless directed otherwise, never hold the breath during the exercise and always work to keep your breathing smooth and even.

We recommend beginning each training session with some breathing and finishing with some breathing and massage. We will be describing some of the core massage techniques later on in this book.

The book is divided into chapters on each of the main areas of training. Though, of course, there is often considerable overlap so these topic headings should only be taken as rough guidelines. Always strive to be creative in your training, use these ideas as a starting point to develop your own exercises.

Just a last mention again to always train safely and with the care of your training partners uppermost in your mind! Okay, let's begin with the Core Exercises.

CHAPTER TWO
CORE EXERCISES

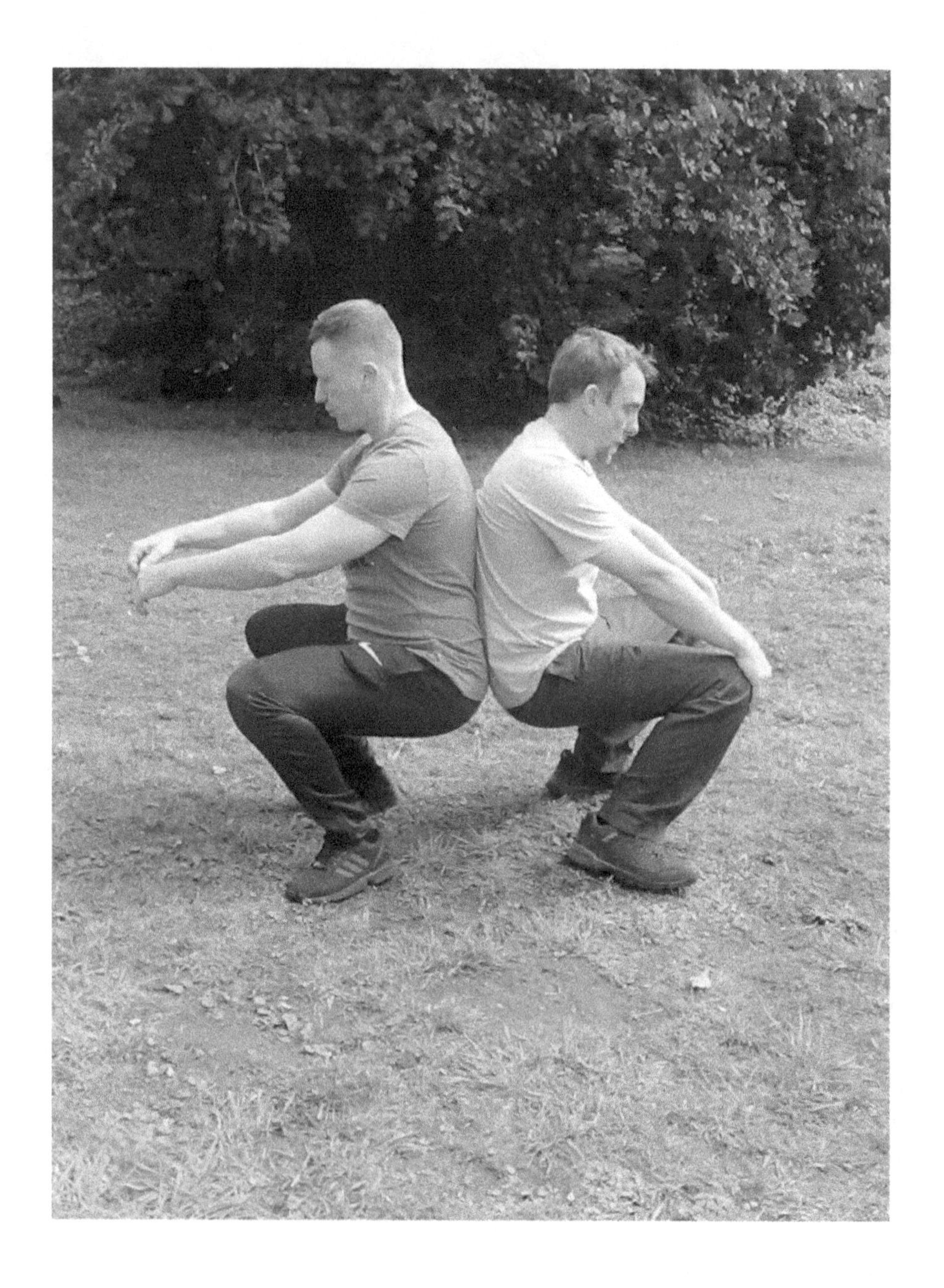

CORE EXERCISES

By Core Exercises we mean the squat, push up and sit up/leg raise that are the foundation of our exercise. With the Core Exercises, there are three ways in which we may interact with our partners.

HARMONISE
SUPPORT
OPPOSE

We will examine each briefly in turn then see how we apply them to our exercise.

Harmonise means that we synchronise our movement/breathing together. So we work at the same speed, the same movement, the same direction. Typically we will work while maintaining contact but not always.

Support means we provide our partner with a stable, or sometimes less stable, platform from which to work. In effect, we are acting as a piece of gym equipment.

Oppose means we apply resistance to our partner's movement or try, in some way, to impede what they are doing. This may be with direct force, or maybe with more subtle methods. It is very easy in most cases to prevent the other person from moving at all by applying an amount of force. However, this is not the point of the exercise, we need to provide just enough force to allow our partner to move but with some difficulty.Let's look at some basic ways we can apply each of these to the Core Exercises.

PUSH UPS

HARMONISE
Get into push up position next to each other, shoulders touching. Partner A (PA) initiates the movement. Go down, then rise up, with the appropriate

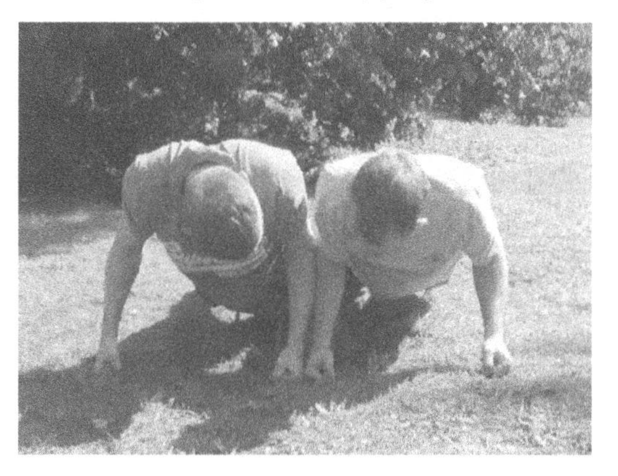

breathing. Partner B (PB) must match the movement and breathing with their own. Once you are into the movement you will find there is less "leading and following", both work together.

SUPPORT
PA gets into push up position. PB holds and lifts the ankles to waist height while the push ups are performed. So the job of the holder is purely to provide support.

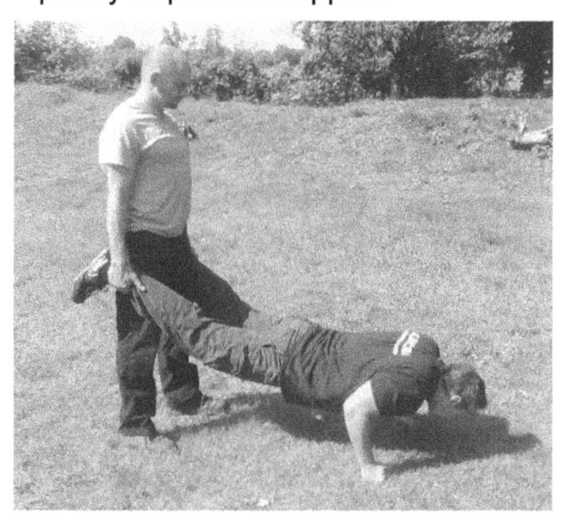

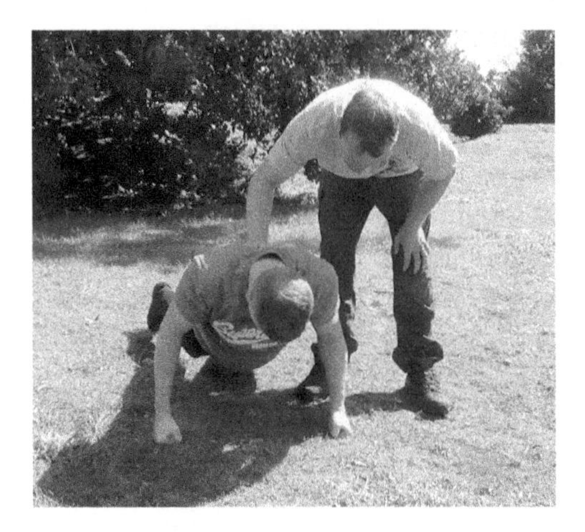

OPPOSE

PA performs push ups while PB applies some downward pressure to shoulder, body, head, etc. PA can either try and flow around the force or work to push directly against it. One will develop relaxation within the movement, the other will develop strength. In each case, the amount of resistance should be measured

SQUATS

HARMONISE

Stand back to back. As with the push up, PA initiates the squat, then both

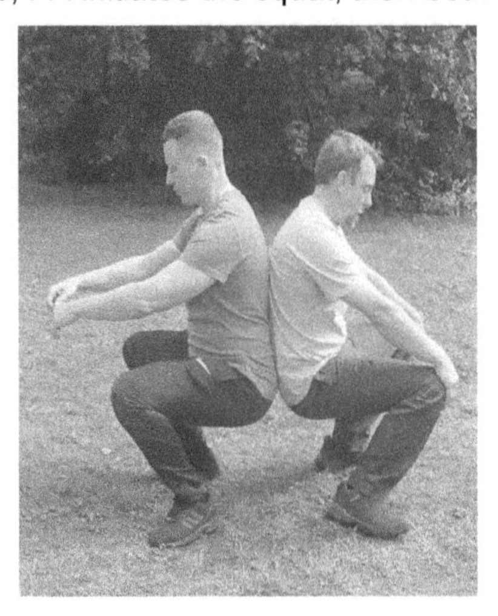

harmonise movement and breathing.

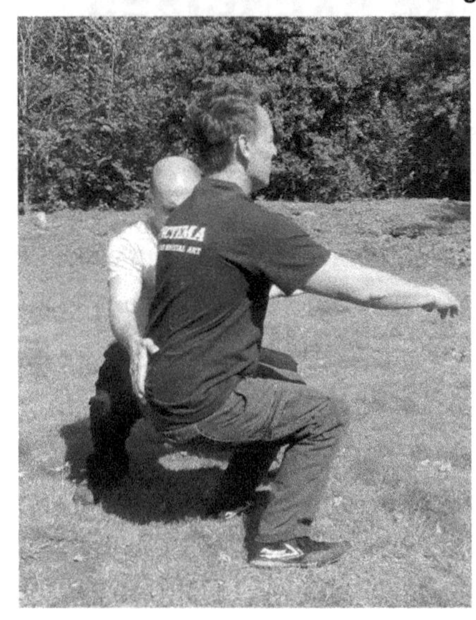

SUPPORT

PA squats. PA places a palm on the chest and lower back. As PA squats, PB supports the structure, helping PA to maintain good form throughout. PB can also move down with the squat.

OPPOSE

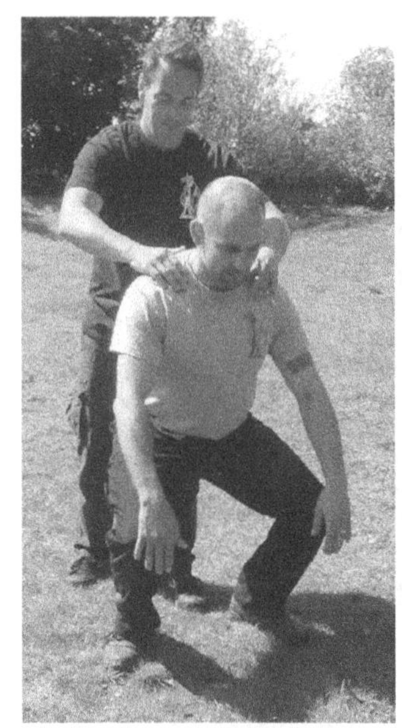

As PA performs the squat, PB applies downward pressure to the shoulders. Again,you can work to move around the force or go directly against it.

SIT UPS

HARMONISE

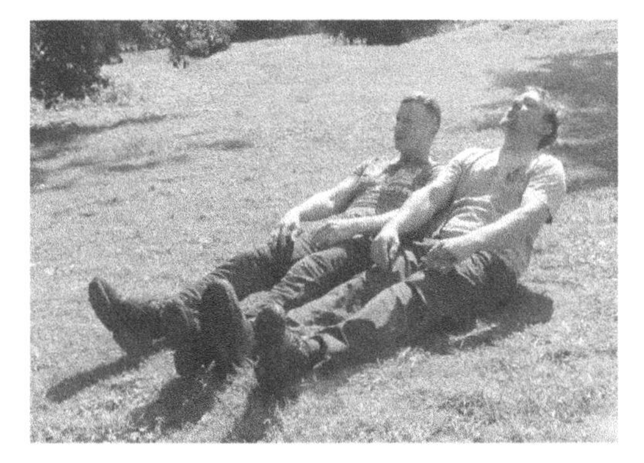

Lay side-by-side and, as before, PA initiates the sitting up, then both synchronise breathing and movement.

SUPPORT

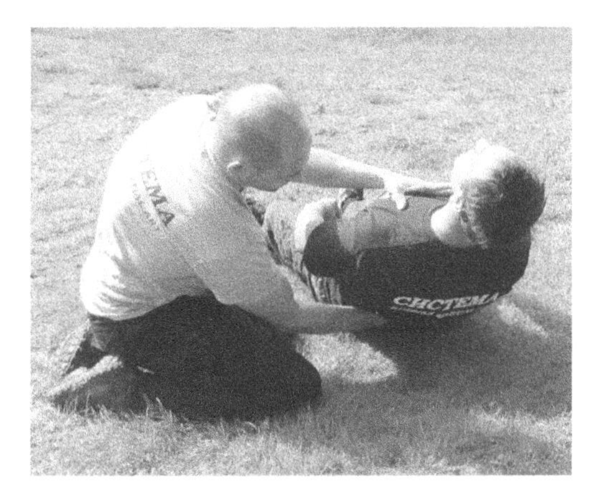

As with the squat, while PA performs the sit up, PB supports the back

OPPOSE

From the same start position, as PA raises, PB applies pressure to the shoulders, torso, etc. Once again, flow around or go through. Be light with the pressure to start, as this is a more challenging position from which to work against resistance!

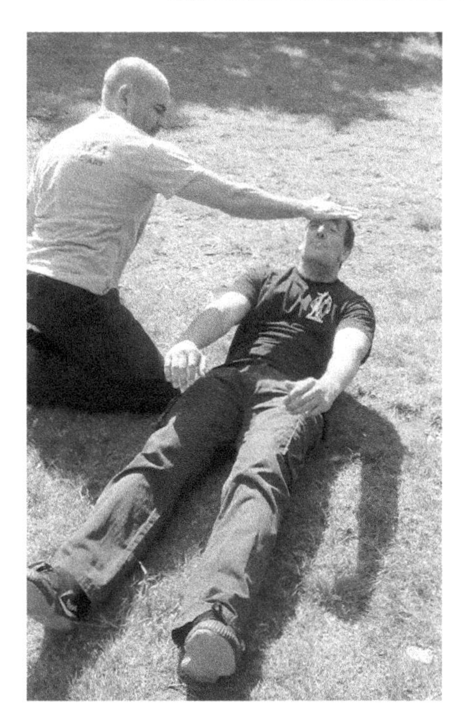

LEG RAISE

HARMONISE

As before, PA initiates the exercise, then both synchronise breathing and movement.

SUPPORT / OPPOSE

PA performs the leg raise. PB either supports the legs or applies pressure to them

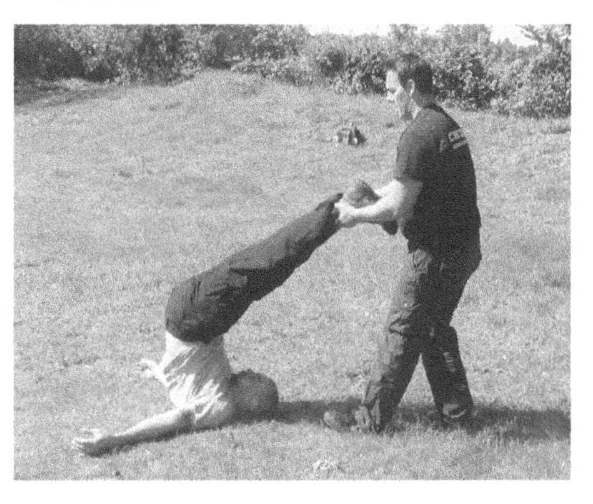

I hope this clearly illustrates the three principles with the Core Exercises. There are countless variations we can perform in pairs with these exercises, let's now look at a few ideas.

PUSH UPS

PB raises the feet as before. This time, though, they move the feet around. This can be changing the height or position of the feet, or move them

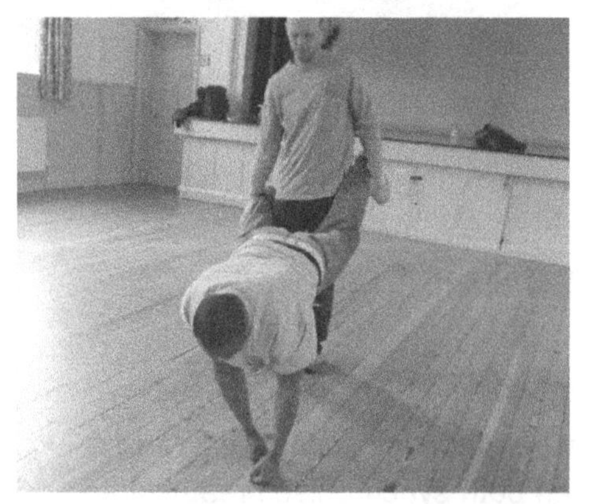

forward or back, as in "wheelbarrow" push ups. For another variation, raise the feet are raised to a point where PA is virtually in a hand stand position. Do the push ups from here.

PA lays on their front. PB places their hands on PB's ankles and does push ups. PB can also raise and lower the lower legs.

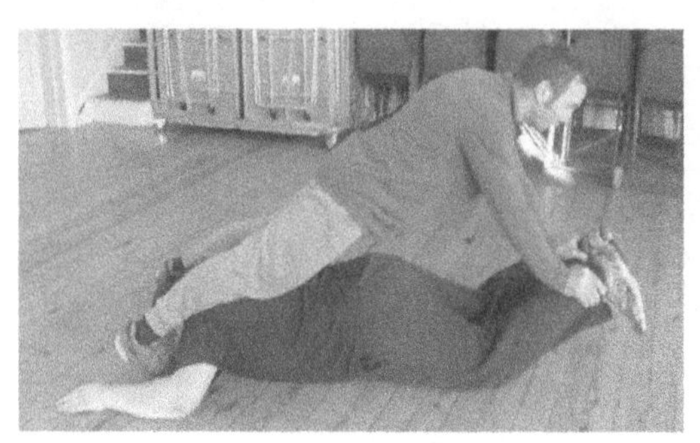

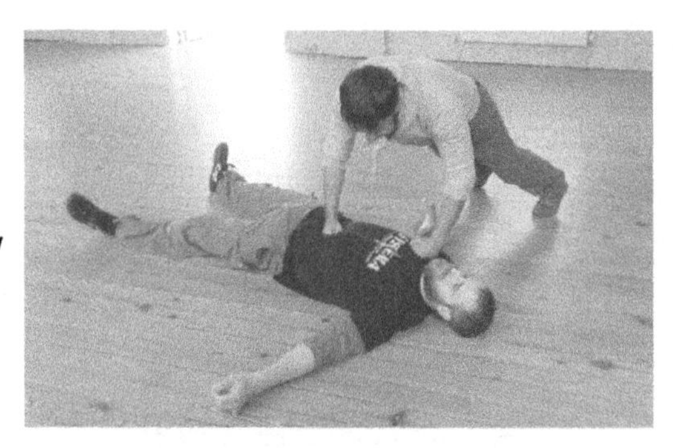

PA lays on their front. PB places their fists in different places around the body and does push ups. The supporting partner can either apply local tension under the fists, or can try to relax under the pressure.

Partner A performs a push up. Partner B then moves a hand or foot to another position and the person performs another push up. Repeat!

SQUATS

Partners face each other and clasp hands together, then do normal squats. Giving each other support in this way

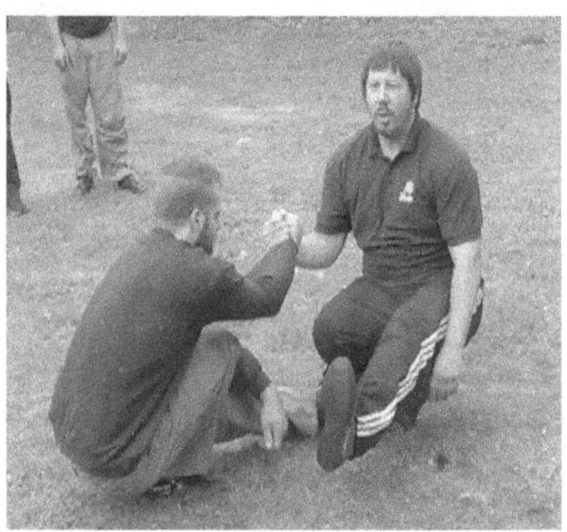

means you can really focus on your posture. For a greater challenge, hold with one hand and try pistol squats.

Try the assisted squat, but very slowly. PB constantly monitors and adjusts PA's posture in order to make sure that the posture is perfect. Once PA is in full squat, keep them there and gradually lessen the support. This is a much tougher exercise than it looks but is very helpful in building the correct posture for squats.

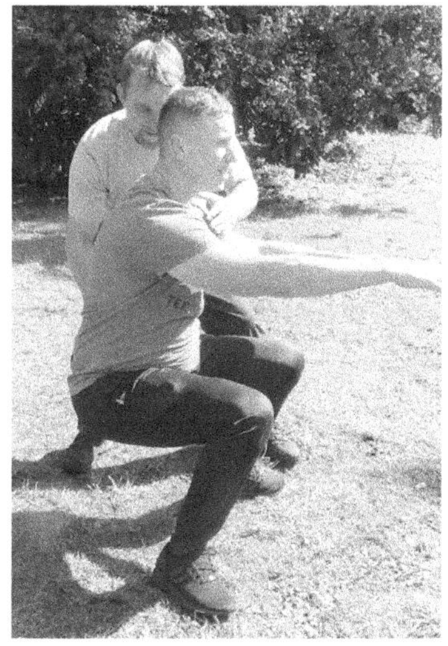

SIT UPS

PA hooks their feet over PB's shoulders. PB hooks their arms under pa's legs for support. From this position performs sit ups. Be sure that PB maintains good form, if necessary a third person can provide support.

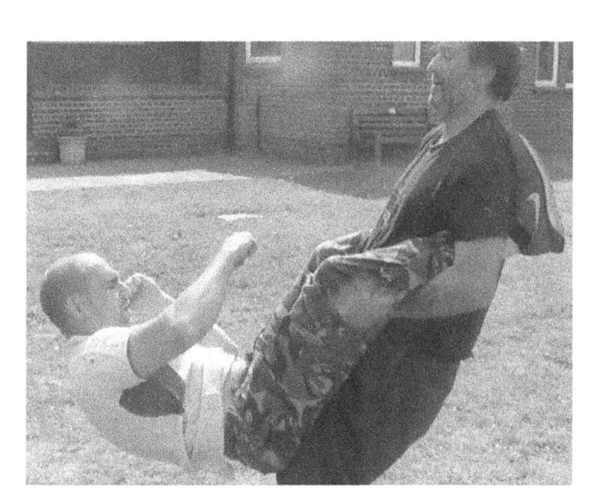

PA lays down with knees raised. PB stands on their feet and PA stands up. Try and perform this in one smooth motion. If you find it difficult, try having PB clasp the knees to begin with. Breathing is key to this exercise!

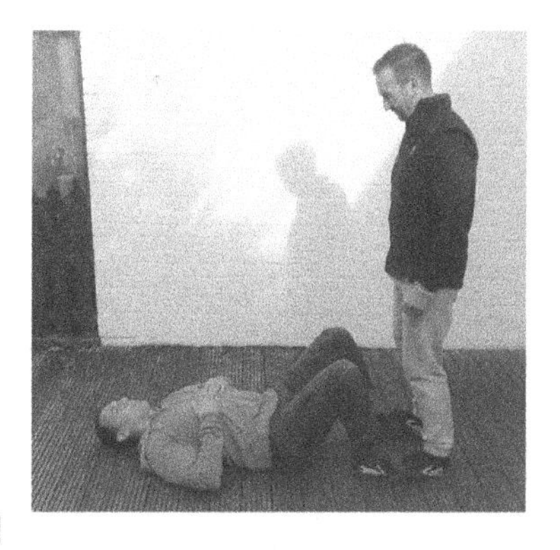

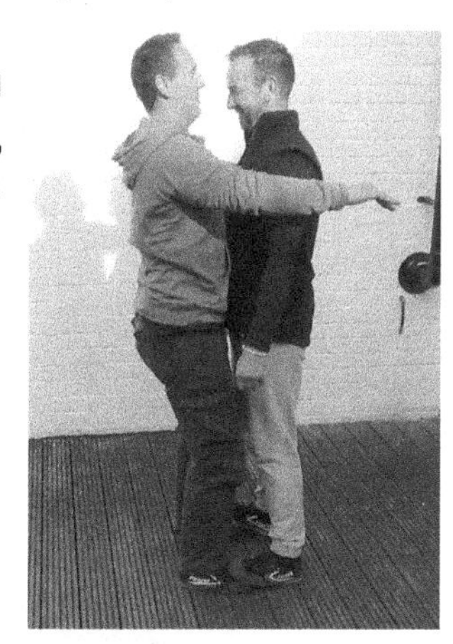

For our final exercise in this section, have PA hold PB's ankles and begins performing leg raises.

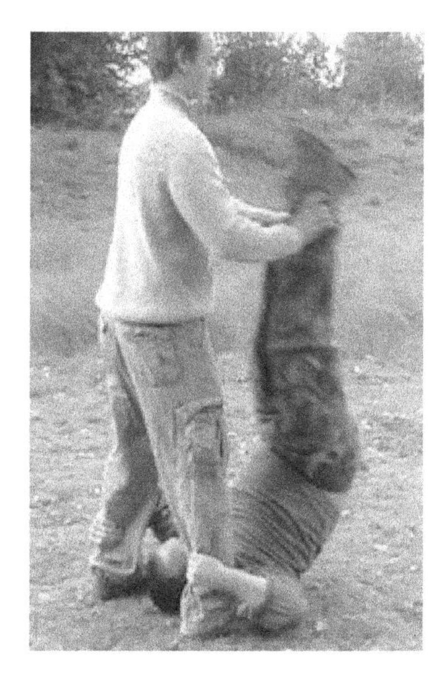

CHAPTER THREE

STICKS

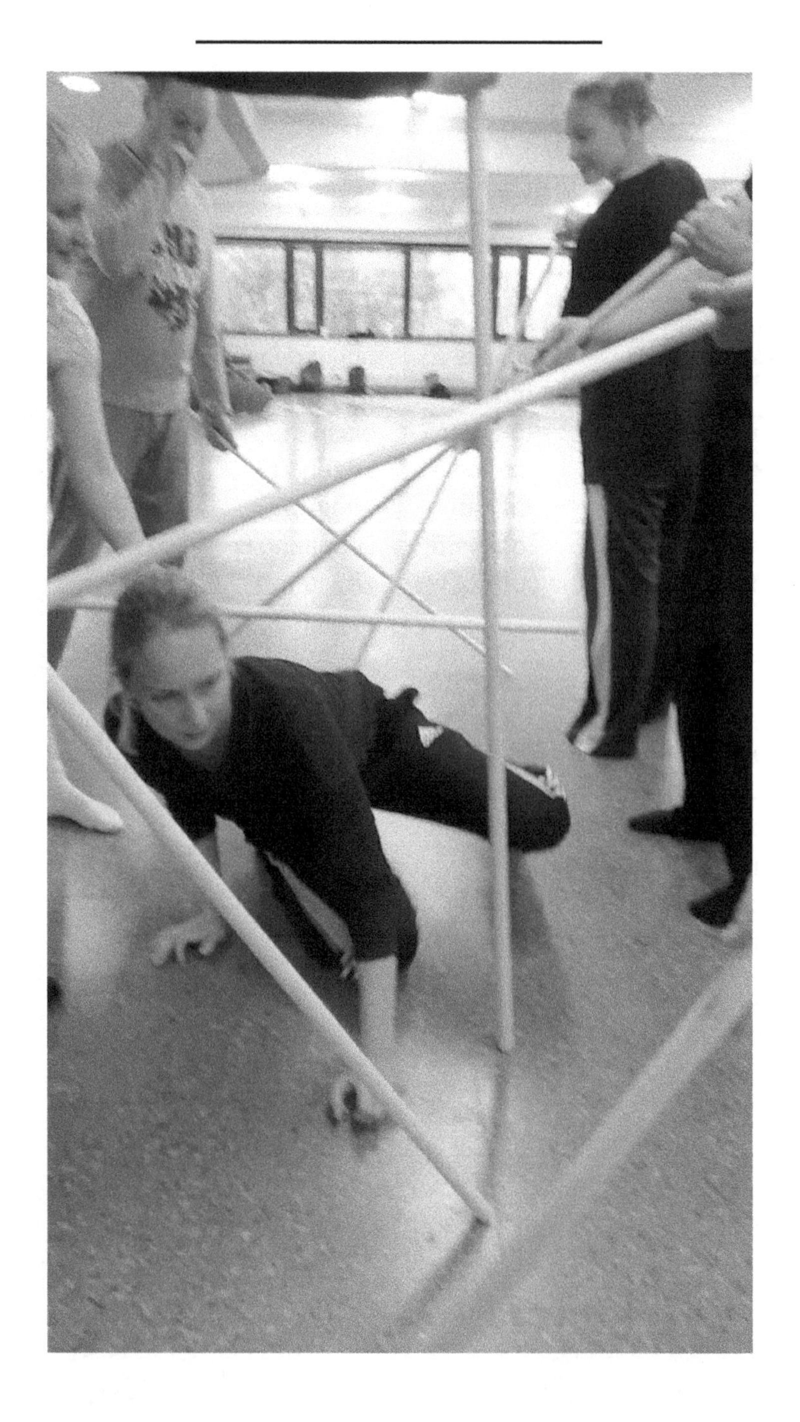

STICKS

As we mentioned in Systema Solo Training, the stick is the most useful piece of training equipment you can have. Likewise for partner training. There are a huge amount of exercises you can do with the stick. They can be broadly divided into strength or mobility exercises. We show you some of each here and we will see some more stick work in future chapters.

Be sure to always use a strong enough stick, one that will bear your weight! Let's start with the Core Exercises and move on from there.

For a push up variation, PA holds the stick across their chest and lays on their back. PB gets into push up position, facing the opposite direction. PA can either hold the stick up in the air while PB does push ups, or pushe the stick up and down while PB does push ups, so both partners get benefit.

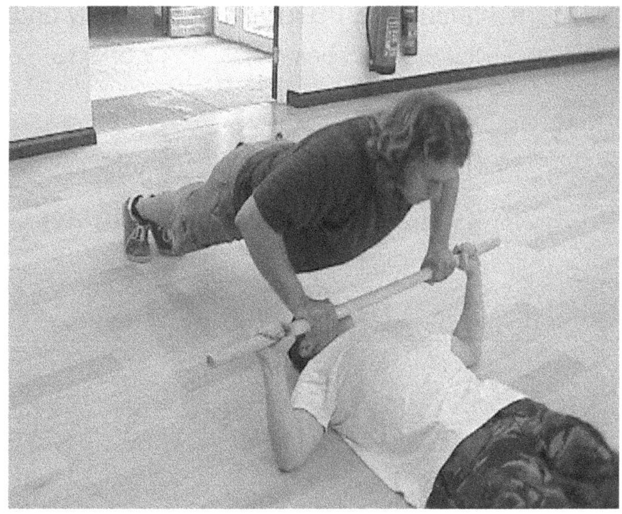

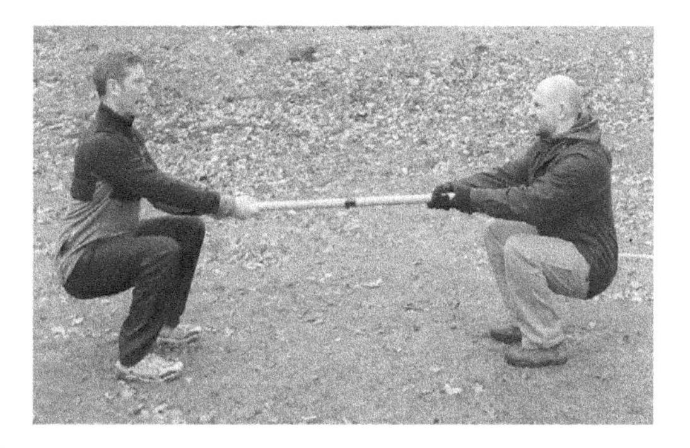

You can try a supported squat with the stick by having both partners hold one end of the stick. As you squat down, pull a little on the stick for support. Try and match each others pull and try to use less and less support as your squat improves.

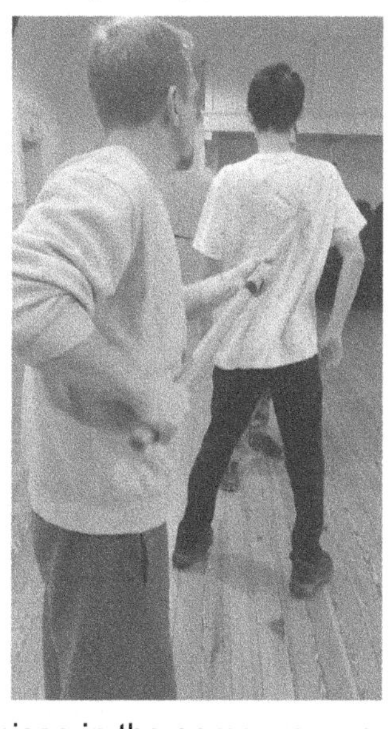

Use the stick in any of the Core Exercises in the same way we used the hand earlier with resistance. PA pushes with the stick, PB does the exercises and tries to flow around it.

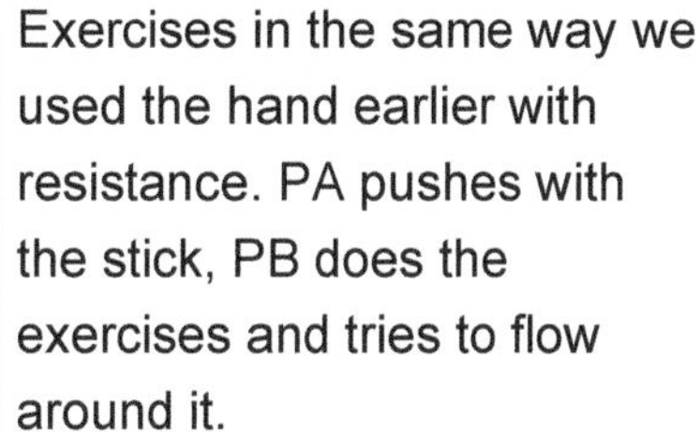

There are couple of very good stick exercises for core strength. Each is weight bearing, so once again be sure you have a strong enough stick! We looked at a

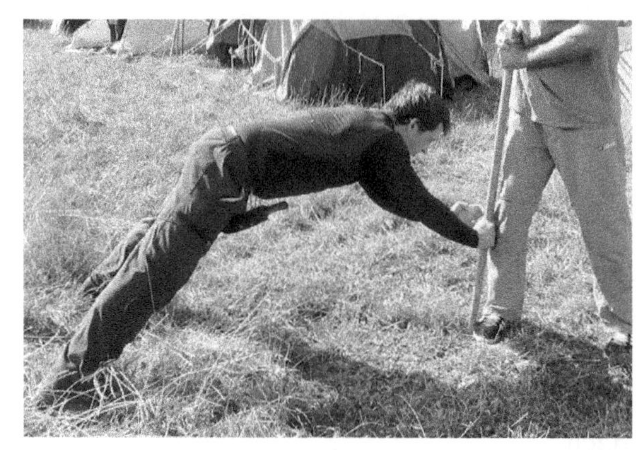

version of the first in the solo training book. Here is the partner version.

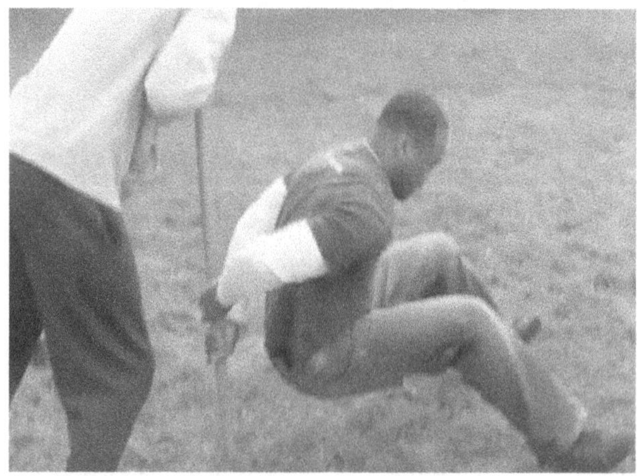

PB holds one end of the stick firmly on the ground. They can reinforce by placing their lower leg against the stick. It is important that the stick is held in place upright.

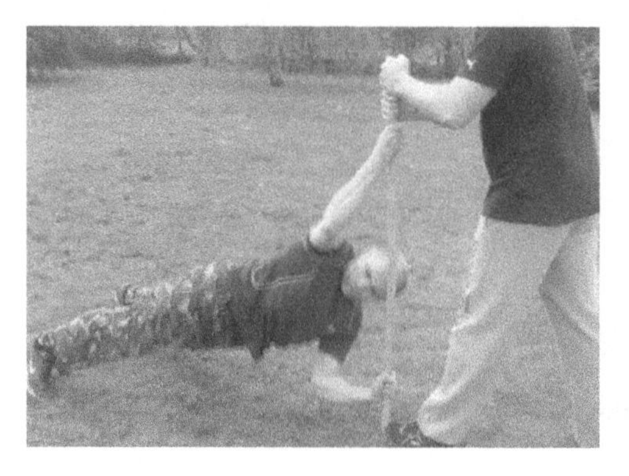

PA holds the stick with both hands and begins to climb up and down it.

As you do so be sure to try and keep the body in alignment, in much the same way as you do in a push up. If working at full stretch is too much to start, then try with your weight on the knees.

For variations, try also doing the climb facing away from the stick. You can also try placing the hands in different positions.

Once you can do this comfortably, try climbing the stick with one hand for a challenge!

For the next exercise, partners start by facing each other with the stick held over PB's head. PA grasps the stick with both hands and PB moves back slightly and lowers the stick slowly. PA works to

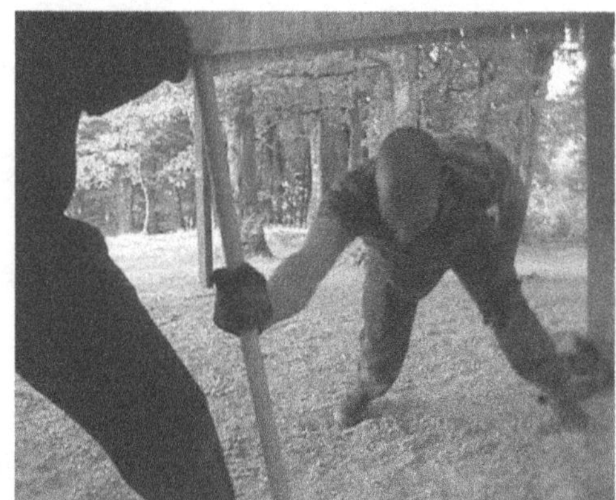

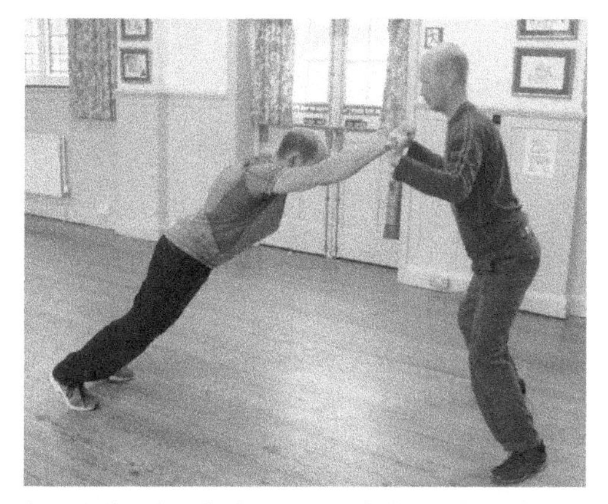

keep the body in as straight a line as possible, keep some tension in the core.

PB should not take the stick too low at first, gauge it carefully. This is another exercise that is much harder than it looks! From the low point, PB lifts the stick back up again. PB should also maintain good posture during the weight bearing part of the exercise.

For the second part of the exercise, follow the same procedure but this time with PA facing away from PB. Be sure

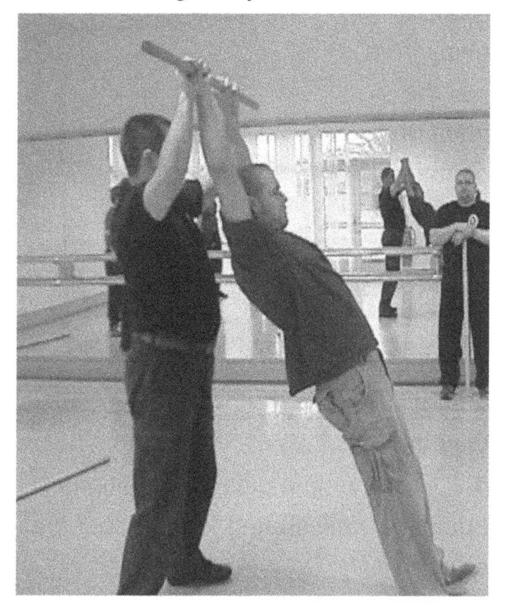

to keep the body straight again, the aim is not to hang off the stick.

We can work grip training and selective tension with the stick with the following routine. There are four positions - partners face each other, stand side on to each side and work back to back. In each position partners

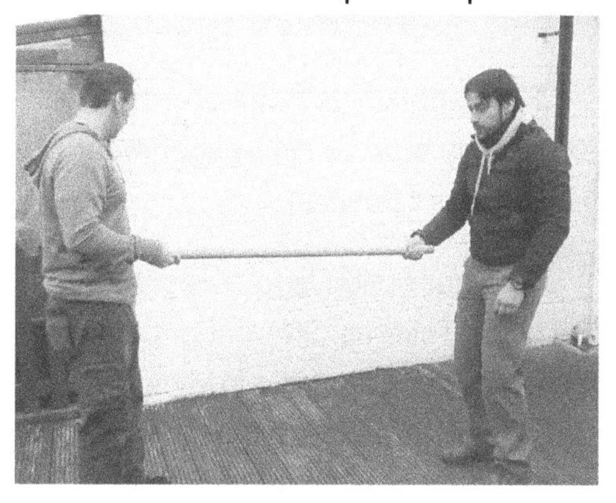

hold the end of the stick and slowly twist and pull. The aim is to build up and maintain an even pull at both ends of the stick. Use selective tension on the fist and forearm, but keep the rest of the body relaxed.

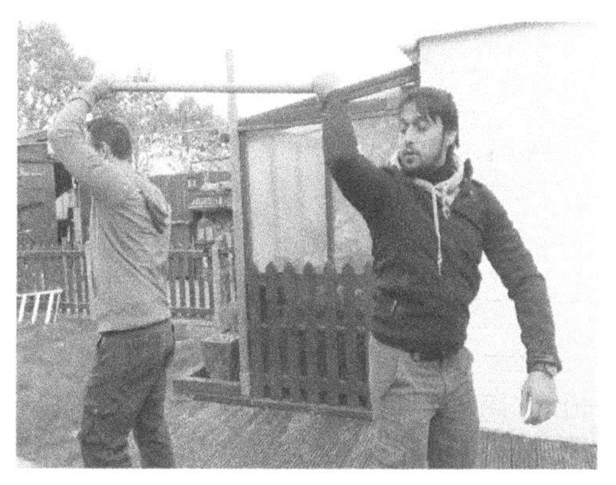

Work each position for a couple of minutes. When facing or back to back you can either use both hands at once or work left and right grip separately.

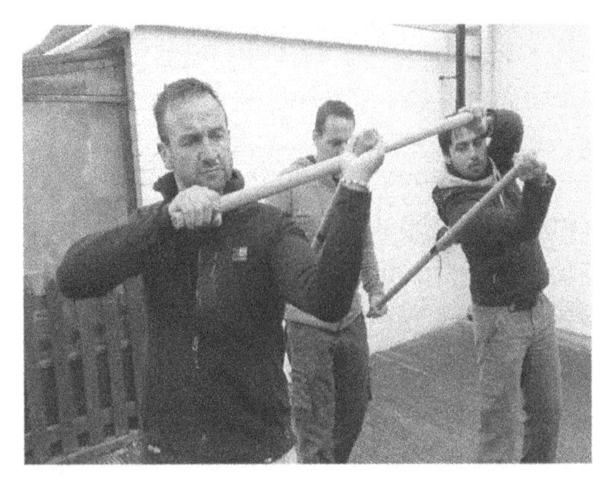

For variation you can also try this exercise in a group and experiment with different positions.

Another option is to "wrestle" with the stick. Take up different grips and move the stick around slowly with tension. Both partners match speed and amount of tension /resistance. Once again, keep the rest of the body relaxed.

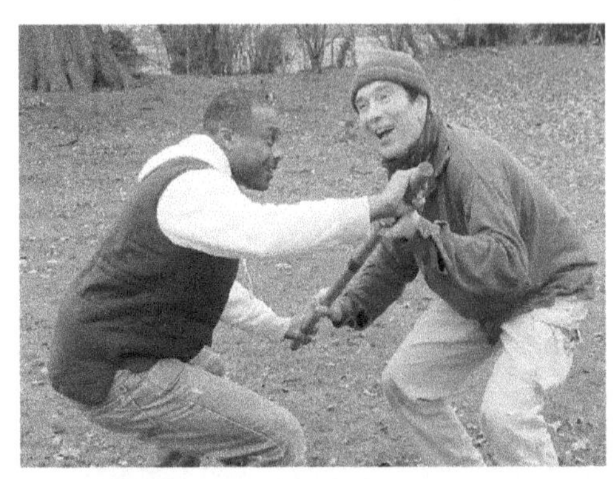

We will return to strength training with the stick later on. Now, let's look at some mobility drills. The purpose of each of these is develop either good joint rotation or full body movement. When working with relaxed movement, particularly when being pushed, be sure to maintain posture and form as

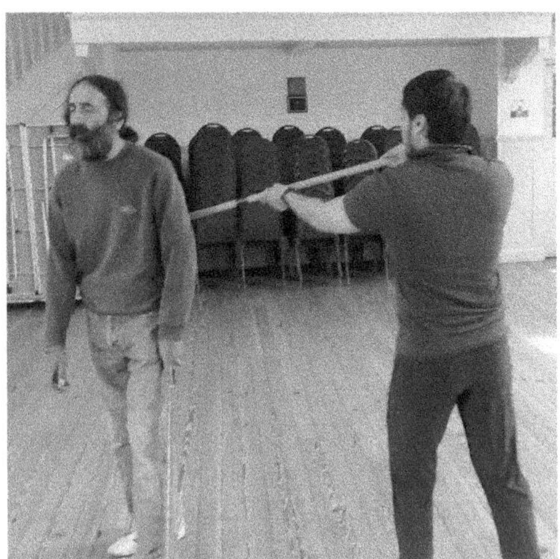

much as possible (unless the drill is to flop/ relax completely.)

To start, PA simply pushes PB with the end of the stick. The push should be firm enough to make the body move. PB responds either by moving the whole body away from the push, or by rotating away from just the point of contact. Exhale as you are pushed.

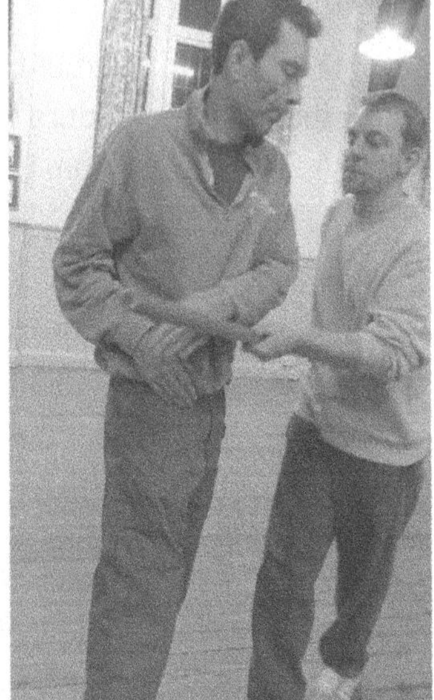

You can easily vary this drill by working in different positions - against a wall, seated, on the floor and so on.

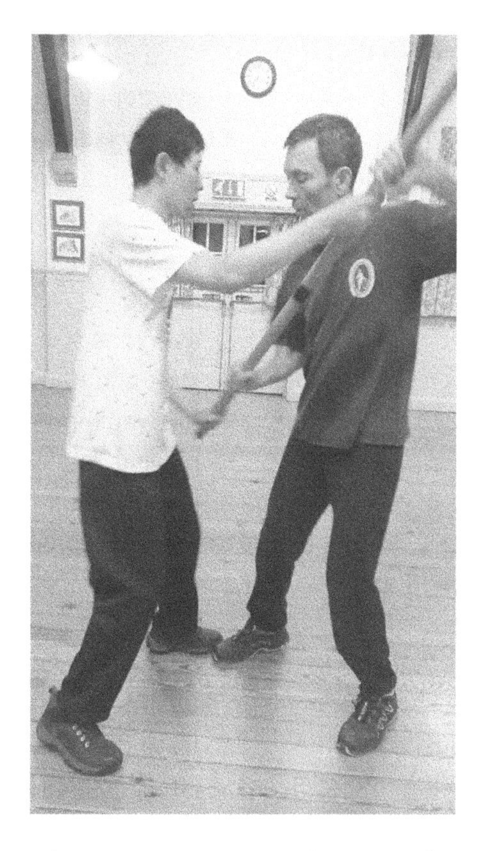

As you progress, try also to work sliding the stick off of the body with the minimal amount of movement.

To work this into a flow drill, then as one partner moves with the push, they also disarm the stick. As quickly as possible, return the push with the end of the stick. Do not "set" yourself in a stable position, but learn to work instantly on taking the stick from the other person.

The stick can be disarmed using leverage, or by working against the hands and arms of the holder. Start in a standing position but also change levels to the floor and back as you progress.

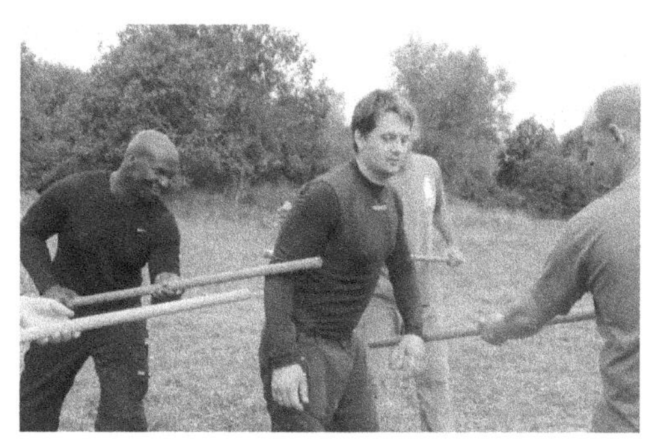

Stick exercises also work well with a group. Have one person stand in the middle and the group all push them with sticks. Don't pause to change over, have the person in the middle disarm a stick wielder in or to change roles.

Of course we can also work with the stick pre-contact. PA swings the stick and PB simply avoids it. You can start with set movements, such as the following:

- downward movement, avoid by moving side to side

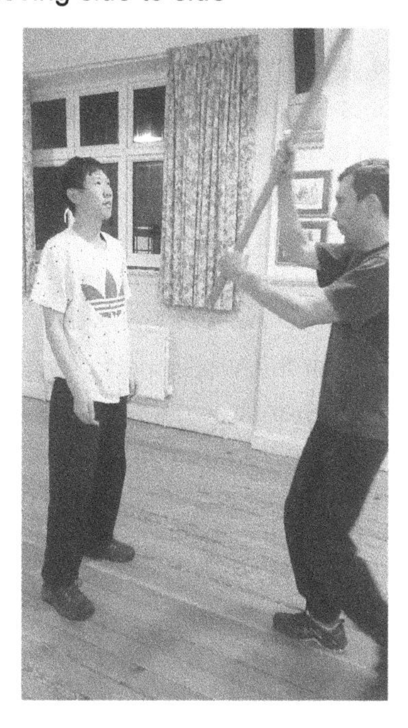

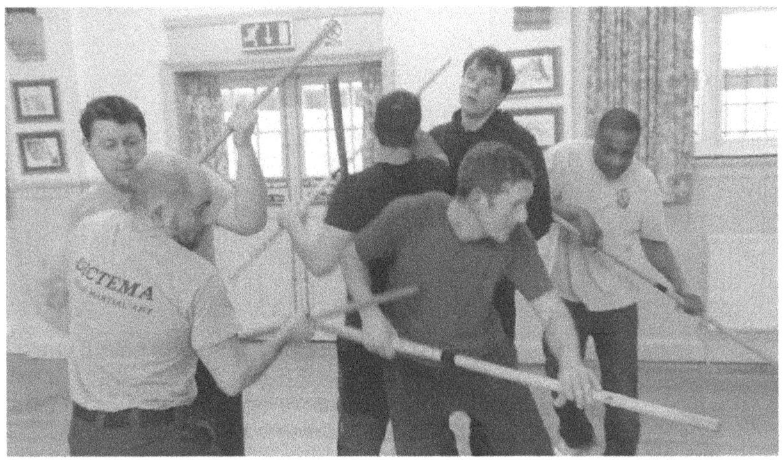

- forward thrust, avoid by turning
- high swing, avoid by squatting
- low swing, avoid by jumping over
- diagonal down, avoid by crouching and moving in.

When moving, keep posture and breathing. It is also a good habit to bring the hands up to cover the head, or as preparation to strike on each movement.

Once you have these basic movements down, the stick holder can now begin to work with more random movements. Always start slow and work with purpose - try to avoid pulling the strike if you think the stick is going to hit. Obviously it is best to use a lighter stick for this work and to start slowly. If you want to work at full speed, try using bamboo sticks tied together, plastic piping or similar. You can then work full tilt without fear of injury.

As with the contact drills. We can work stick avoidance in groups. So have one avoider vs three stick wielders, for example. In class we sometimes like to give everyone a stick and have the whole group moving and avoiding at the same time - be sure to use appropriate speed and levels of contact.

Another variation is to have one stick wielder in the middle. The group have to avoid and also try and move in to “tag” the stick holder. If a person gets touched with the stick on the way in, they have to move back to the edge of the training area.

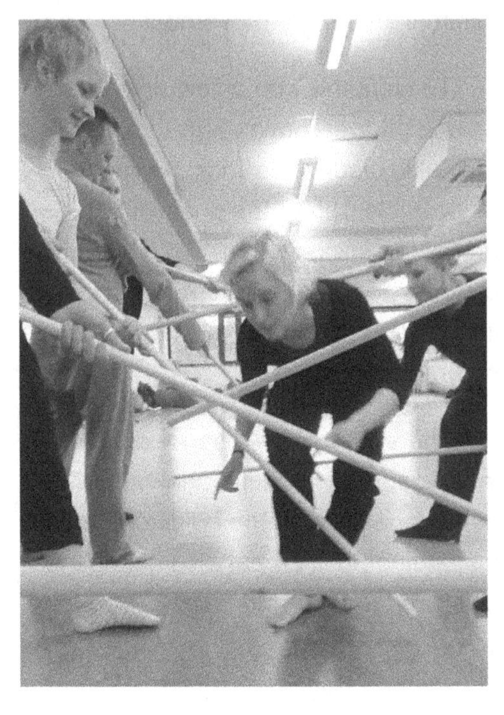

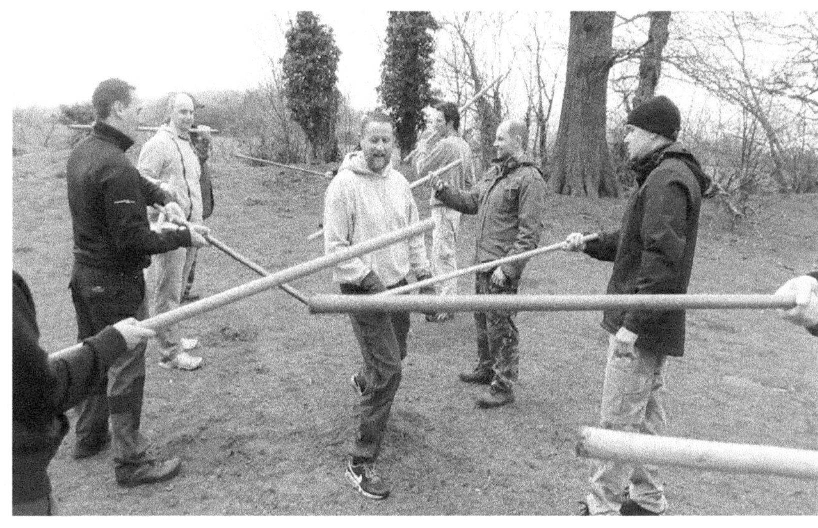

We can also work gauntlet drills with stick avoidance. The simplest is for the two rows of people to position then hold sticks in place. Each person takes it in turns to travel the length of the line without touching any of the sticks. You can start of with the sticks in quite easy to avoid positions and work up to more complex positions.

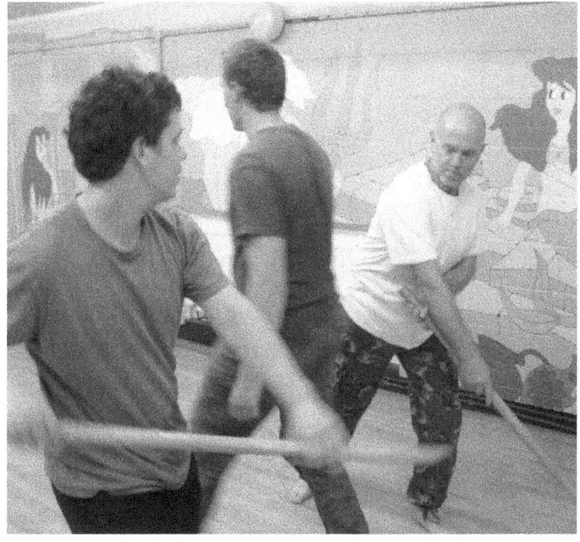

The aim again is to move through the space as freely and smoothly as possible. Try not to stop and think about it too much, part of what you are learning to do with this drill is to evaluate and move into spaces as quickly as possible.

From here, the stick holders can next move the sticks. Each person works in a fixed pattern at first, ie one movement repeated over and over. Each person again has to get the length of the gauntlet while avoiding contact with the stick. If you do get touched, roll it off and move on.

After this, you can try the same drill with random movements of the stick. Exercise caution again, use lighter sticks if necessary.

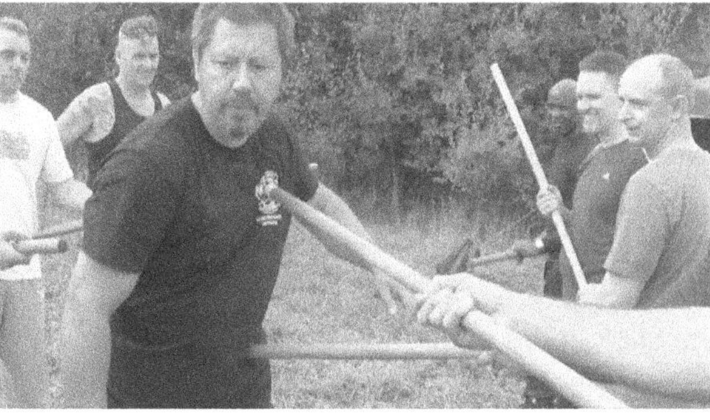

The final level for this sequence of drills is to try each again with the avoider blindfolded. Obviously there is much more work from contact this time but we have had some quite surprising results, with people avoiding even random sticks with some practice. Listen to your inner voice!

From big movement, let's now take a look at a great stick exercise for joint rotation and flow. It is a two part exercise and both parts start the same way and follow the same procedure.

PA faces PB and rests a stick on PB's shoulder. PA should hold the stick lightly in place for the first exercise. The stick is going to be moved through the following sequence:

Shoulder to shoulder
Elbow to elbow
Hip to hip
Knee to knee
Ankle to ankle
and then back up again.

In the first part, PB moves the stick in the sequence above with their arm, hand,

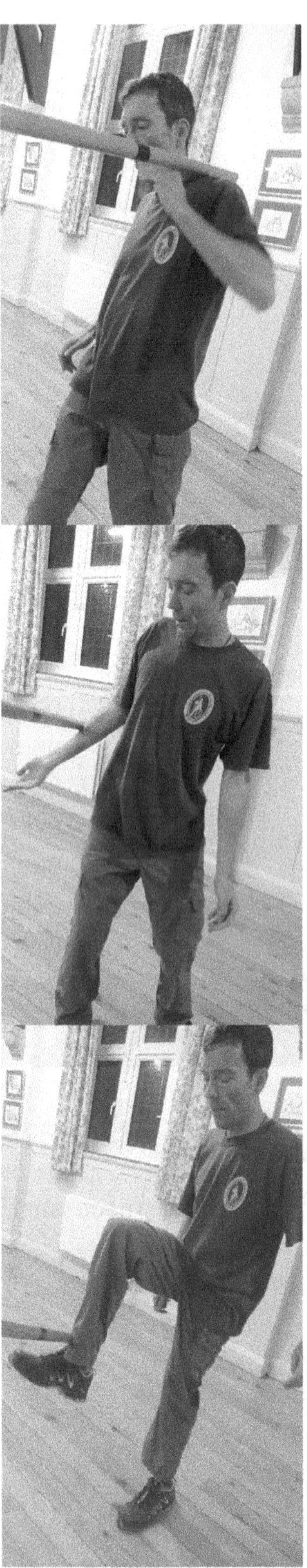

or however else they wish too. Do each movement a few times, then PA moves the stick to the next part. So, for example, the stick rests on the shoulder, it can be lifted over the head to the other shoulder and back again a few times. Following this, PA moves the stick to rest on the elbow and so on

PB has to maintain contact and an element of control over the stick throughout. Follow the sequence down, then back up for two or three times.

The second part of the exercise has the same setup and sequence. However, the difference is that this time, PA must hold the stick firmly and try not to let it move. So PB now has to move around the stick, following the sequence again. This time you will find you have to move your feet at times to accomplish the task.

For both parts of the drill, keep movement fluid and light. Be creative in moving around the stick, part of this is about problem solving!

Once you have tried this drill with the stick you can put it into all sorts of work against a person. Think, for example, as the arm as a stick. Have your partner come in with a grab and work how you can either move the arm, or move around, whilst maintaining contact with your partner.

This ties in with a simple physical fact when dealing with an incoming force. There are four options available:

1. We move completely out of the way
2. We move/deflect the force
3. We move around the force
4. We deflect the core while also moving around it.

You can work this concept against sticks, grabs, kicks, punches and so on. If you ever find yourself getting stuck in any of those situations, come back to this stick drill for a "reset". You can, of course, find other variations in the basic drill too. Change the start positions, work seated, hold something in the hands, try working with two sticks and so on.

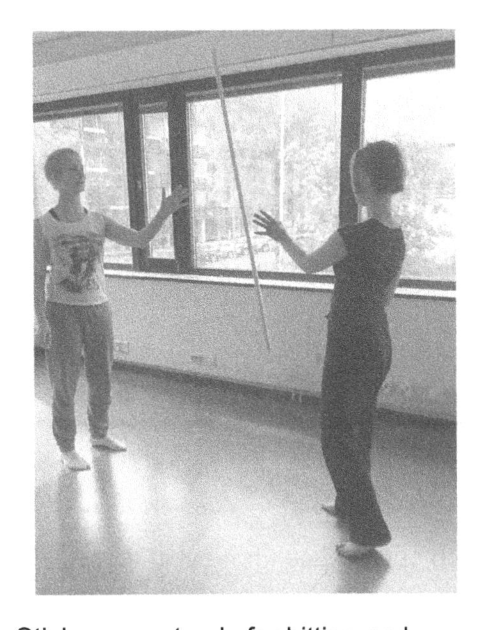

Sticks are not only for hitting and pushing! Let's take a look at another series of exercises that involve catching and throwing. These exercises are primarily concerned with developing peripheral vision, awareness and ease of movement while carrying out other tasks. You can also substitute the stick for tennis balls, or any other suitable object. Needless to say, you need to have a decent

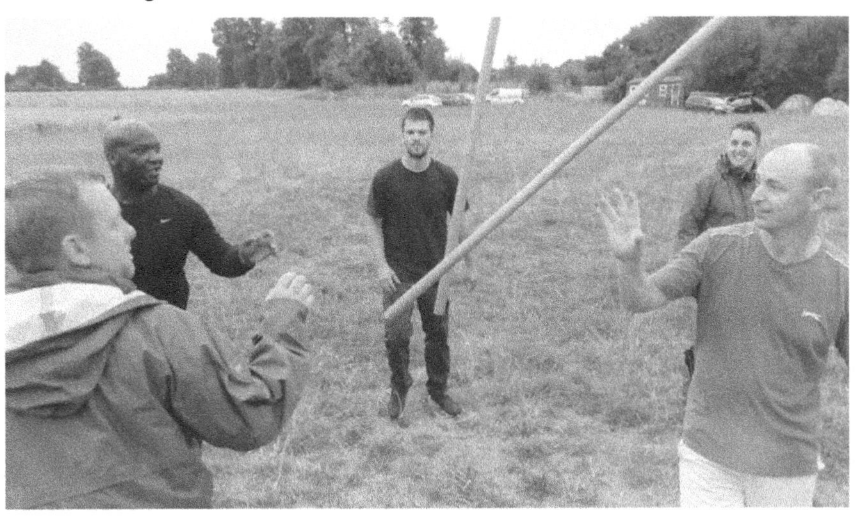

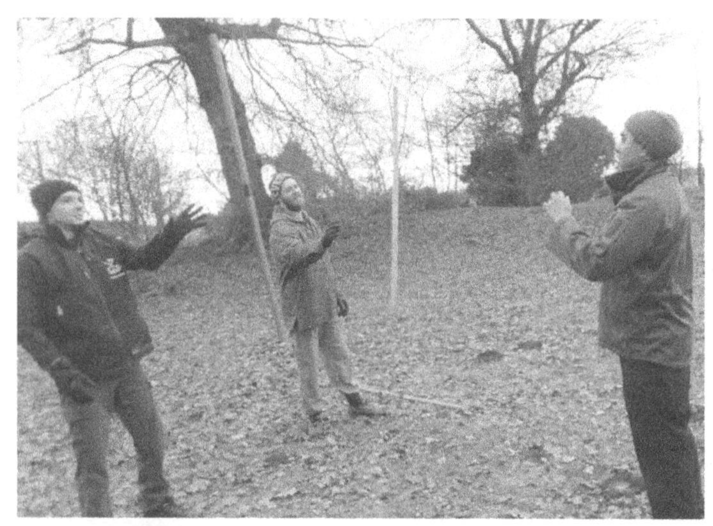

For the next stage, work in groups of three. You can also add an extra stick. Once again, be aware of how you pass the stick to your partners. Be mobile too!

If you have a larger group, try this. The group stands in a circle, a few feet apart from each other. You begin with one stick, which is thrown from person to person in the circle. You throw to anyone, it should be random. Try and get used to throwing the stick as soon as you catch it and do not switch hands or grip.

After while introduce another stick into the drill. Then, after another while, bring in a third. You can go up to as many as you like but, of course, the drill gets progressively harder the more

sized open space for most of these drills.

Stage one is to work and pairs and simply throw and catch the stick between you. Let's establish some base rules before moving on.
First off, you always throw the stick to the person and not at them. Throw in such a way that the stick is easy to catch - ie lengthways on rather than end on!

Start the drill static, then both partners begin moving. When moving, throw the stick to the space you partner is moving into, not where they are.

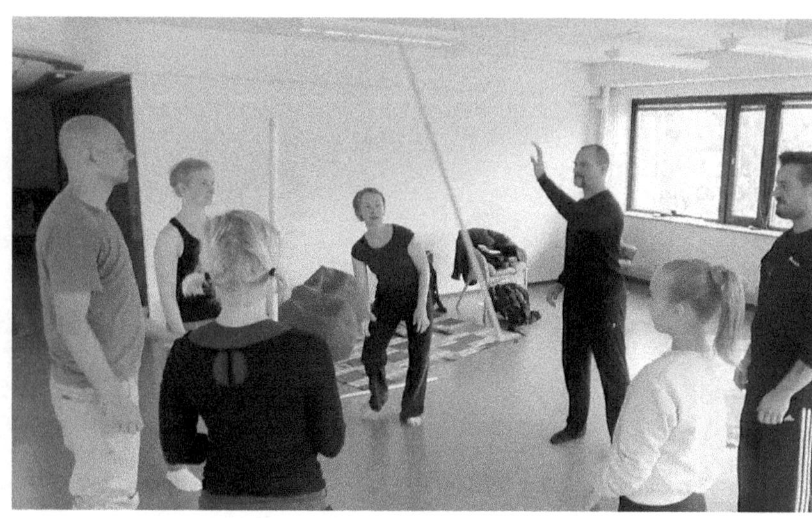

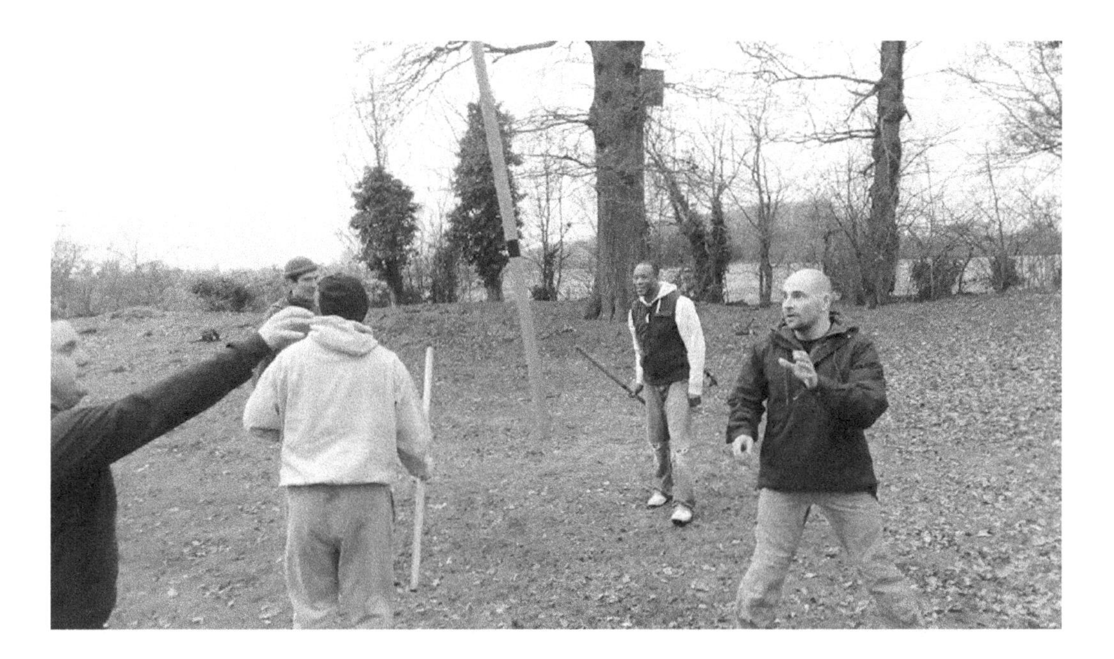

sticks there are. Don't lose sight of moving and throwing well and, naturally, check your breathing and posture.

Now, let's try a variation on the circle drill. You need around half a dozen people. PA stands in place and the others make a semi-circle facing, you need to be around 6-8 feet or so away. We being with one stick again. PA is the "target". The group throws the stick only to PA, who must immediately throw it back to any one of the group.

As before, gradually introduce more sticks into the group to increase the level of challenge. One other rule in this drill, if sticks are dropped it is up to the group to retrieve them, PA does not move from their position!

Once you have a handle on these drills, go back to the first circle drill, but this time everyone is walking around. Now you need to be aware 360 as sticks can come from any direction. Start with a single stick and gradually add more in again.

These are simple drills and seem like a bit of fun, which they are, but they do have some very positive and concrete benefits. We find that when run at the start of a session, they get everyone into a good, calm mindset. They also sharpen up reactions considerably.

On an application level, we can think of the catch as a deflect and the throw as a punch. From here it should be easy to see how these drills can be worked into to developing counter-strikes and similar.

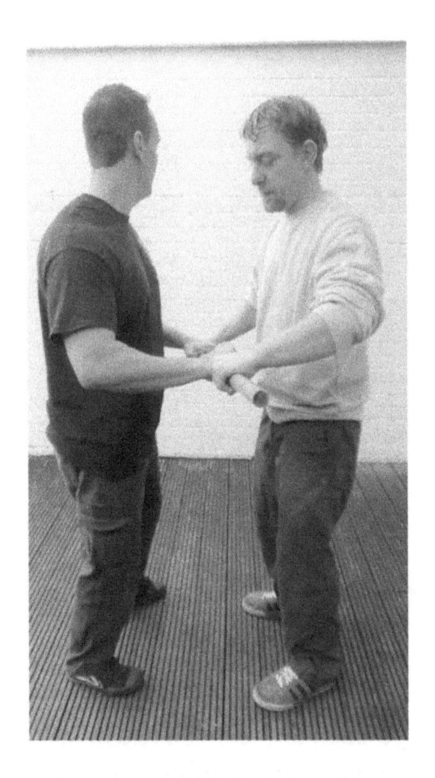

Let's go back to some partner drills for strength building. Begin with a simple movement. PA holds the stick at waist height and pushes it forward. PB provides steady resistance.

From here PA can work into the usual "gym-type" weight training movements - curls, lifts, etc.

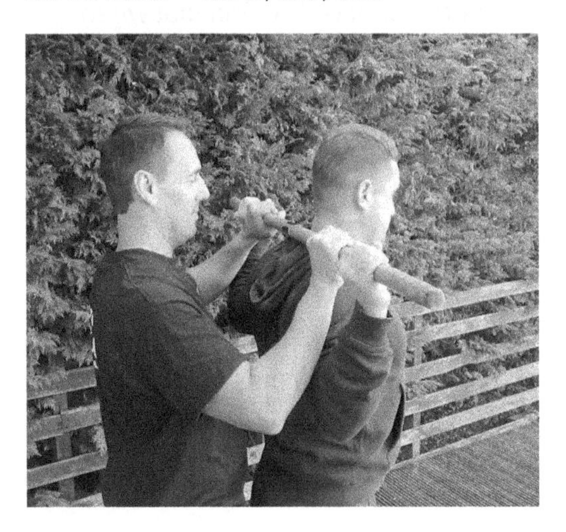

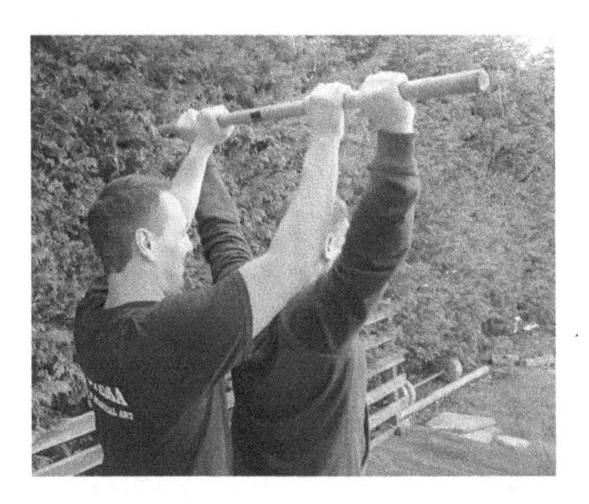

At first PB should apply "smooth" resistance but after a while they can introduce more "shakiness" into their resistance. This prevents the exercise from becoming too fixed.

Once you have tried the conventional range of movements, begin to experiment with different angles and positions. Of course, you don't have to be standing either, work

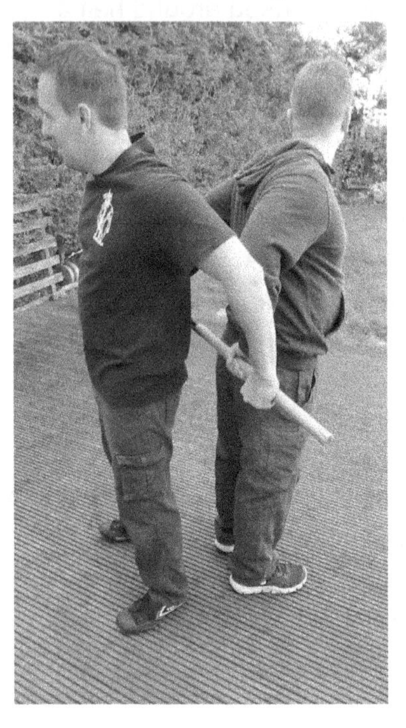

SYSTEMA PARTNER TRAINING

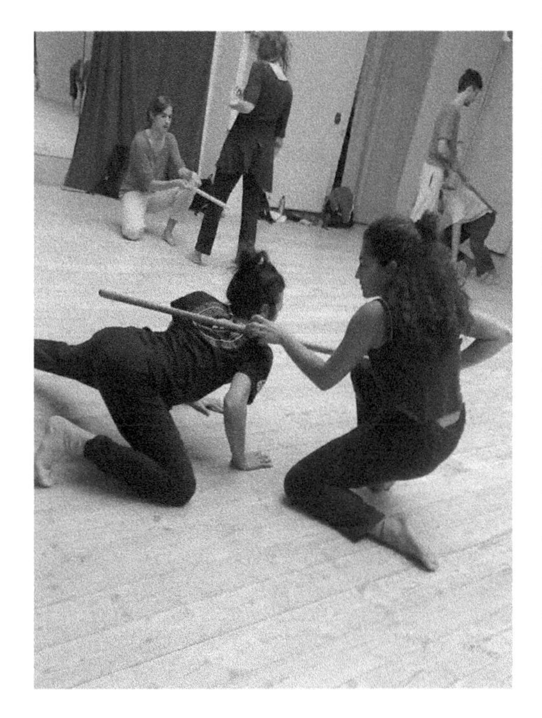

seated, on the floor and so on. You can also add in another person, have one partner hold each end of the stick for added resistance and instability

After strength training it is always good to do some movement to get rid of any excess tension. So let's finish this chapter with some mobility drills.

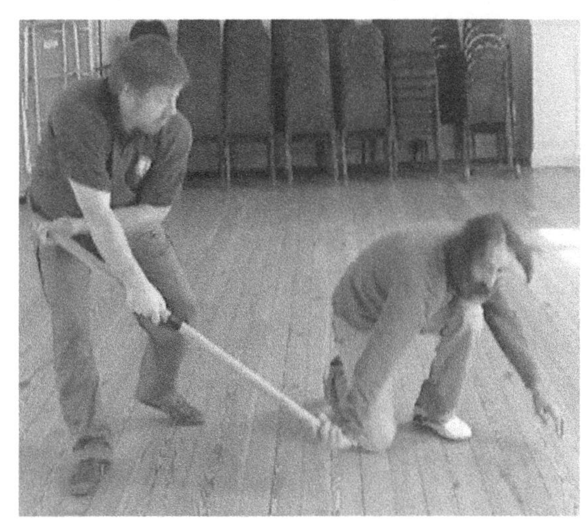

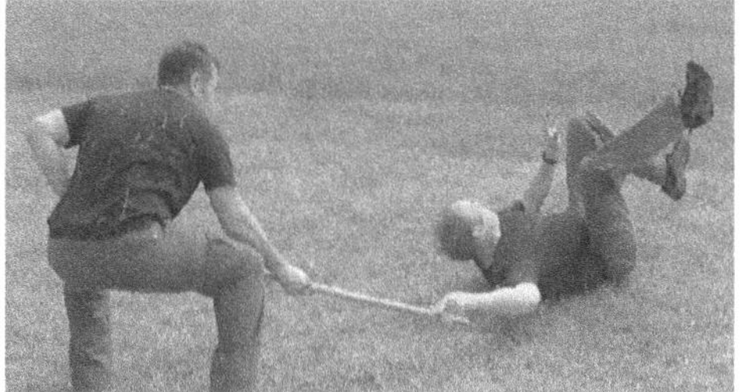

PA holds the stick a distance of off the floor. PB's job is to move under the stick as smoothly as possible. Obviously, the nearer the stick is to the floor, the more difficult the task. You can also work against a wall and, of course, try the same thing with more than one stick holder

For the last exercise, PA holds one end of the stick with one hand. PB moves the stick about in various directions. PA's job is simply to keep hold of the stick. PB should make simple movements to start, becoming more complex and level changing as the drills goes on.

If you want to take this drill to the next level, PB works with more vigorous and more circular movements. You can then work up to PB actively trying to throw PA via the stick. This drill is also a good opportunity to PB to learn about throwing techniques, particularly the footwork required. As a general rule, for any kind of takedown or throw, if you are having difficulties then check your footwork, the solution often lies there!

CHAPTER FOUR
STRETCHING

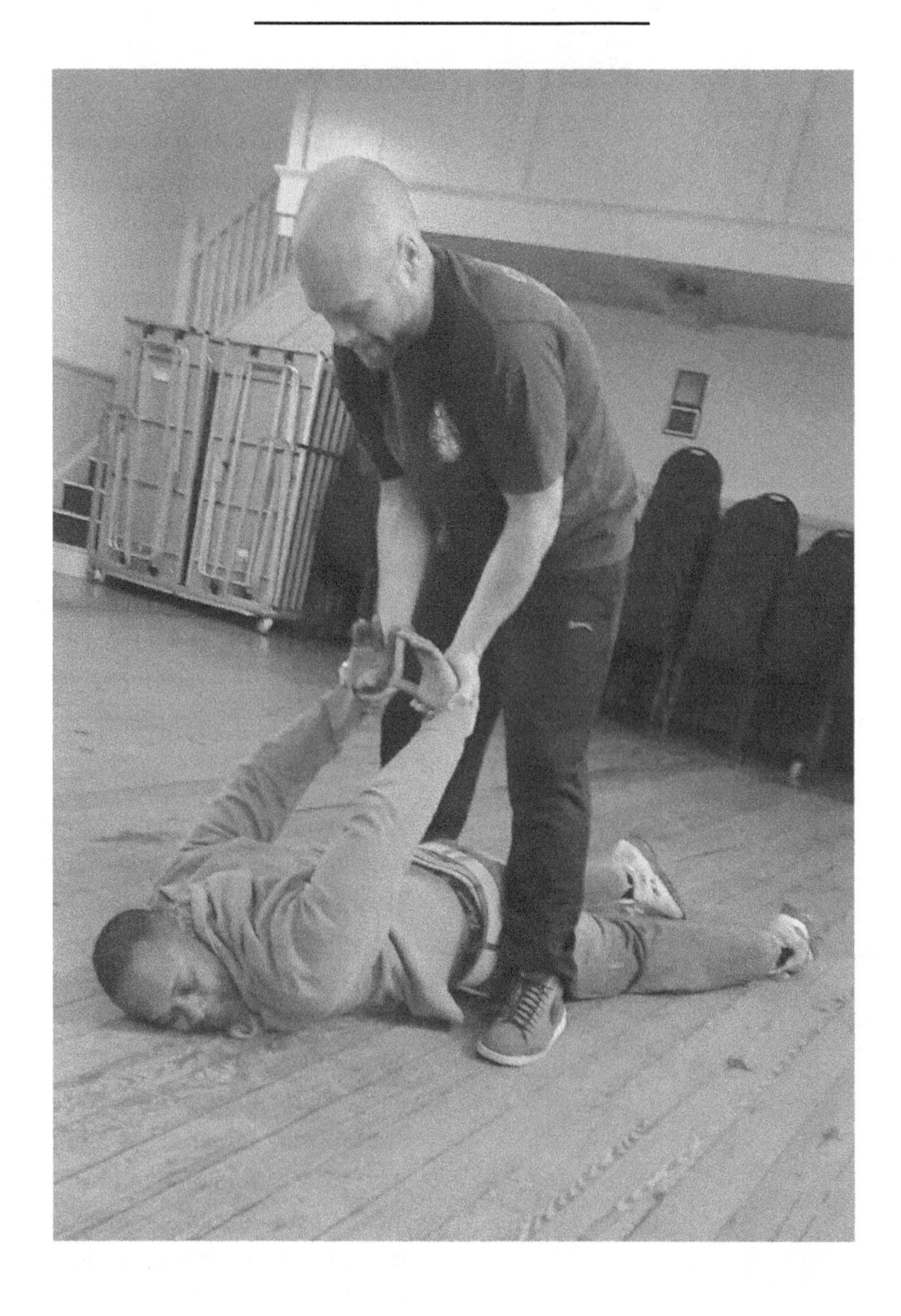

STRETCHING

As we discussed in Systema Solo Training, our approach to stretching is based on relaxation and releasing the "inhibitor reflex". This can occur when our body moves into an uncomfortable position and the muscles tense in order to protect the body from injury. Unfortunately they often tense well before the point of possible injury and so our range of motion is restricted.

To overcome this reflex, we work to the point of first tension. The stretch should then be held static at that position and the relevant muscles tensed on an inhale. Try and hold the breath and tension for at least thirty seconds. Then exhale and relax. You should find that the relax muscle will now "stretch" further. Work to the next level of tension and repeat.

Obviously there is a point beyond which we should not go and there is nothing but potential injury to be gained from forcing out body outside its natural limits. However,we should strive to work to our maximum capabilities in order to develop both good health and freedom of movement.

When working solo we are obviously aware of our own body. When stretching with a partner we must exercise that same sensitivity to our partner. Listen to their breathing, watch and feel for signs of discomfort and tension. Never rush your partner and never, ever move them quickly while under tension. At the end of each stretch allow the body to move slowly back to its neutral position.

From the other perspective, having a partner assist us with a stretch means that we can often go beyond the levels of working solo. Give your assistant feedback, tell them if you need less or more of a push. If you feel any sharp pain or discomfort tell your partner to stop immediately. Remember to work with your breathing, never try and muscle through a stretch. Above all, take your time and work in small increments. Better to think long tem gain than short term glory.

Almost every part of the body can be stretched and the exercises here are by no means exhaustive, but they will give you a good start, as well as a base to create your own ideas. Once you have the basics down, be creative!

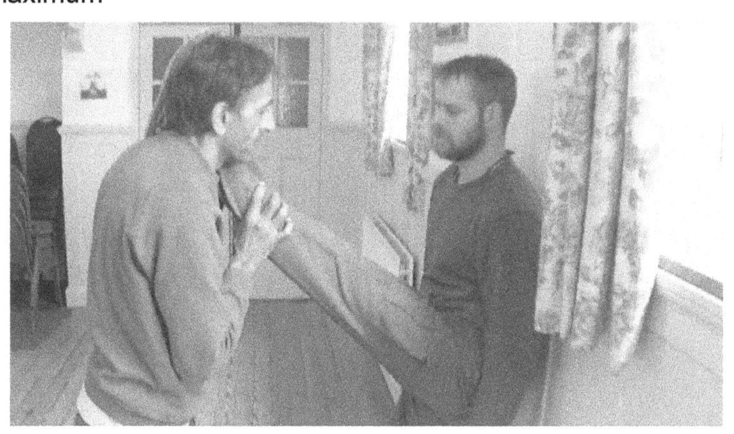

We will split our exercises into upper and lower body. And start with some basic twisting.

PA stands or lays down. PB holds a wrist or ankle and begins to slowly twist and rotate the limb. You can also do this exercise in groups,with up to four people, one on each limb.

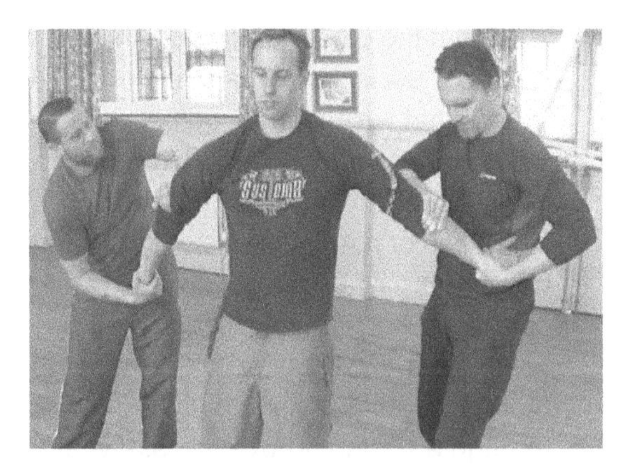

PB holds PA by the upper arms and slowly lifts and rotates their shoulders. PA next raise their arms from the elbows in a "hands up" position. PB holds inside the elbows and slowly pulls PA's arms back. Repeat the same movement, this time PA pushes the palms of their hands together behind the back.

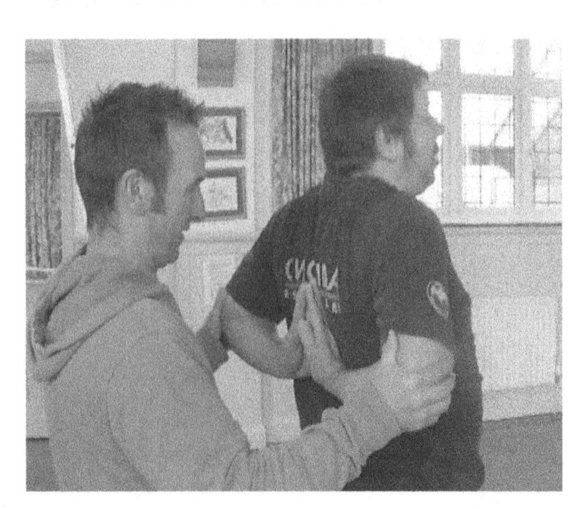

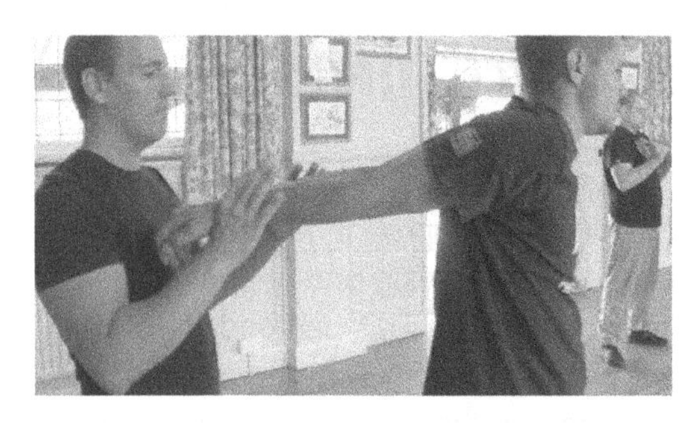

PA stands with hands at sides. PB holds the wrists and lifts the hands up and back. PA should keep their shoulders relaxed. PB now moves the wrists in towards each other. If tension stops the movement, run through the breathing protocol described above. The aim is to get PA's hands touching behind their back. PA can also rotate the shoulders and squat down from this position. When done, PB slowly returns the hands to the start position.

PA stands with hands at sides. PB threads an arm between PA's arms and back, at elbow height. PA inhales, then on the exhale PB squeezes the elbows together.

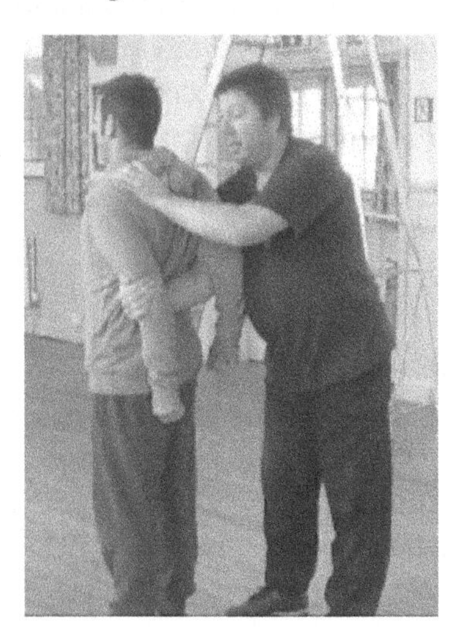

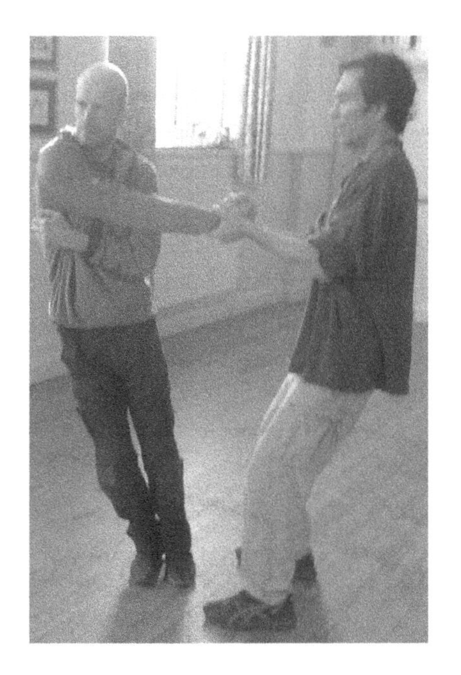

PA crosses their arms across their chest. PB holds one hand and pulls. PA should push the other hand in the opposite direction. They can also lean the body slightly away from the pull. Allow the upper back to open out.

PA lays on their front. PB takes the wrists in the same way as the standing

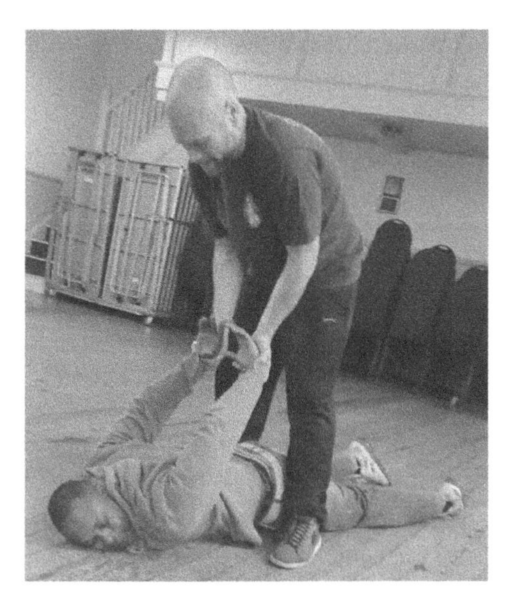

exercise previously and works to bring PA's hands slowly together.

PA lays on their front,with hands behind the head. PB squats and places their hands under PA's elbows, then

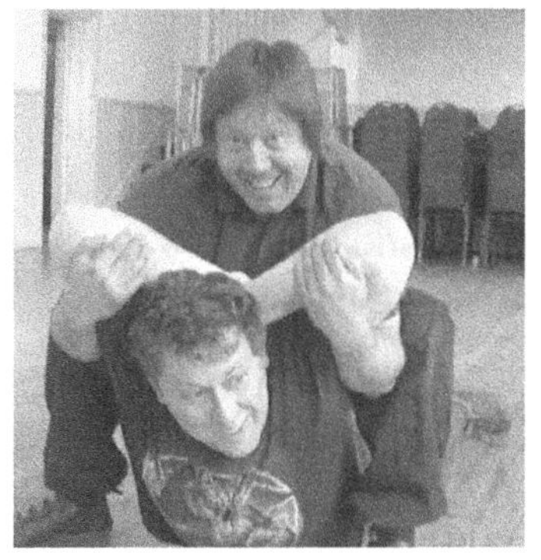

slowly lifts. Take to the end of the movement, then slowly return PA to the start position, It is best for PA to turn their face to the side on the down move, just in case!

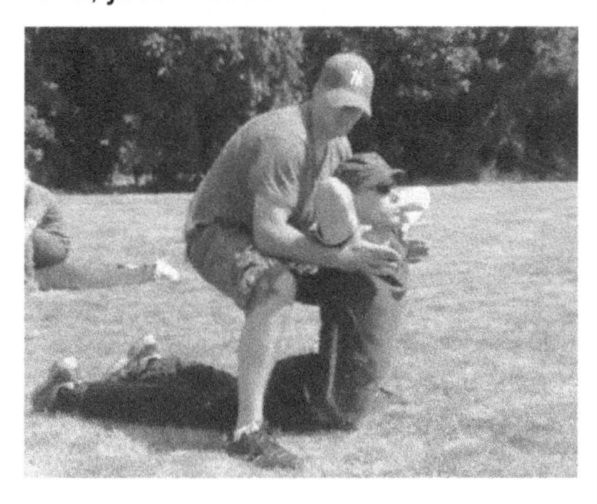

PA lays on their front with hands behind their head. PB holds their

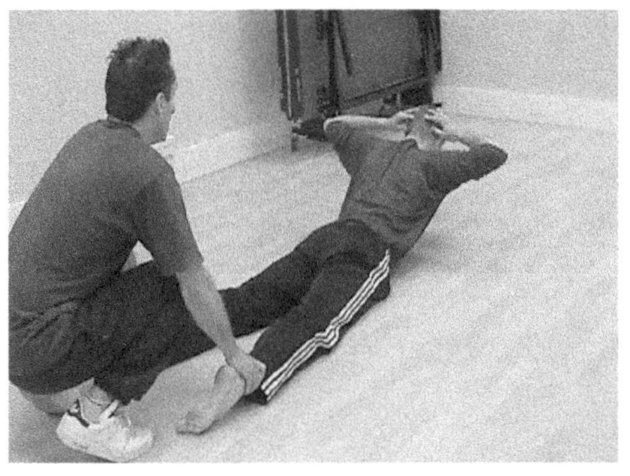

ankles down as PA bends the body up and back.

LIFTS

There are some very good stretches and spinal adjustments we can do by lifting our partner. There are obviously some safety issues to bear in mind before carrying out these drills. First, both partners should have a healthy back. Second, be sure to lift in a safe way, ie using the legs and the body, as you would any heavy weight.

One aim of these exercises is to allow gravity and the body's weight to pull the spine back into alignment. Our spine often kinks slightly out of line and, when it does, the back muscles usually tense in order to hold things in place. Once the spine is realigned, the muscles will relax. This is often the root cause of "everyday" back pains and tension. Obviously any more serious problems should be treated by a medical professional. If in doubt, do not attempt these exercises, the last thing we want to do is aggravate an existing condition.

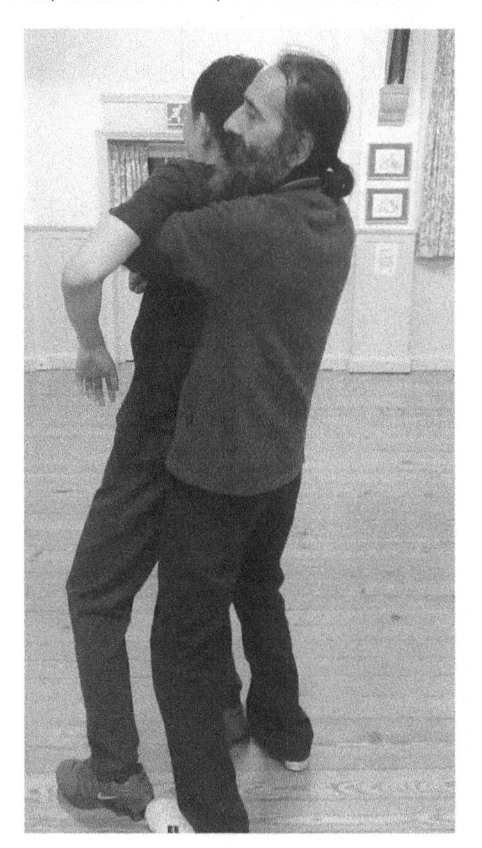

BASIC LIFT

PB stands behind PA and holds them around the chest in a bearhug type position. PA inhales. PB lifts PA and gives them a little "shake". PA exhales on the lift. You may hear / feel a click or crunch in the back, don't worry, this is the spine moving back into position!

There are some variations on this lift. PA can stand with elbows forward. PB now holds and lifts from the elbows, again with a little shake on the lift.

PA places their hands behind the head. PB threads their hands through, in a "full nelson" position. PA now leans back, lifting the toes and allowing PB to take their weight. As this happens, PA squeezes their elbows forward. On the exhale, PB gives a sharp lift, this should release the spine in the neck and upper back area.

For the next lift, the partner is taken up onto the back. Partners stand back to back and link arms. PB now squats down and bends, lifting PA up onto their back. Take care to work from

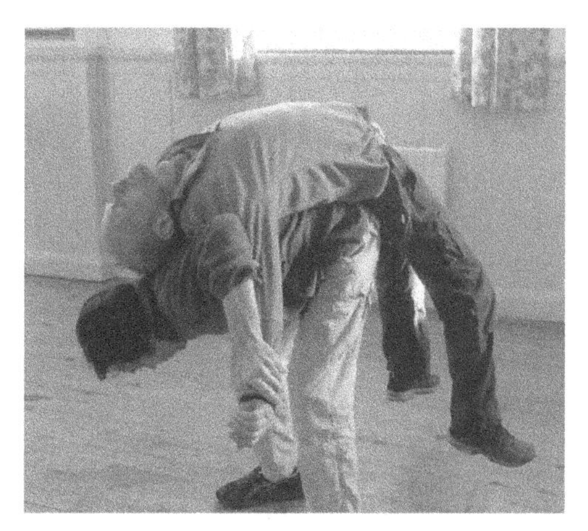

the legs, the lift itself should be a scoop and lift type movement. PA relaxes totally, their arms can be stretched out to the side by PB or pulled overhead. PB squats and straightens to return PA to a standing position.

FOUR WAY LIFT

PA lays on the floor. Four people hold a wrist or ankle. On a signal they lift PA and slowly pull the limbs.

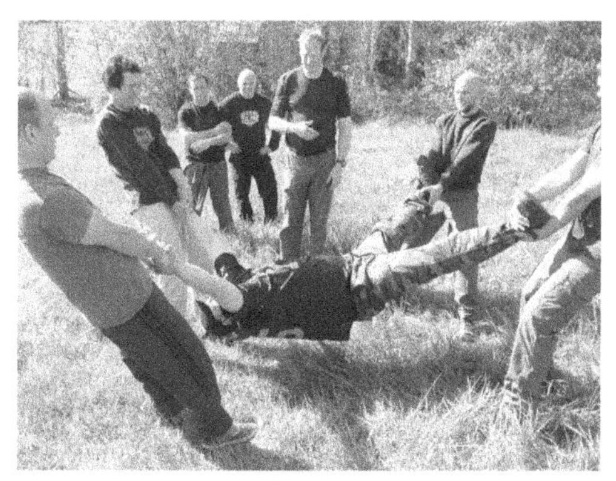

LEG STRETCHES

PA sits with legs outstretched. Keeping the back straight, exhale and bend forward to touch the toes. PB

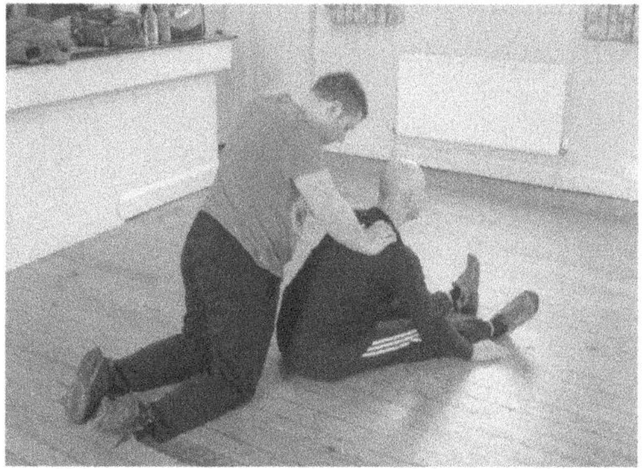

assists by pushing on PA's back.

PA sits with the soles of the feet together. On the exhale PB pushes slowly down on PA's knees.

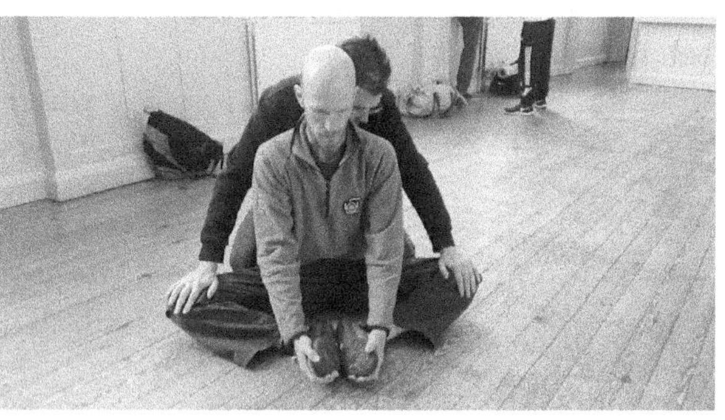

For a deeper stretch, PB can stand on the legs. Be sure not to bounce!

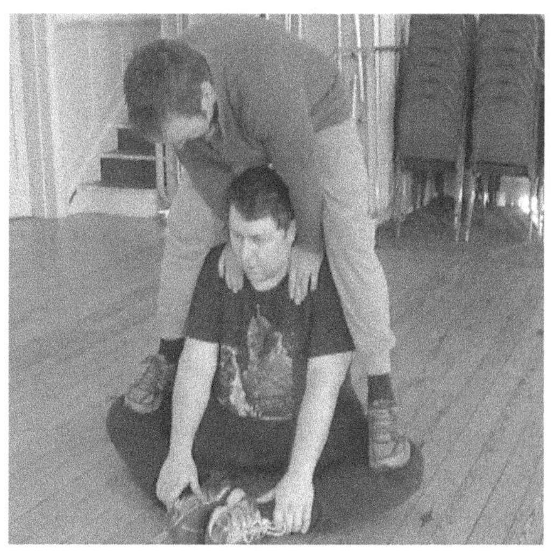

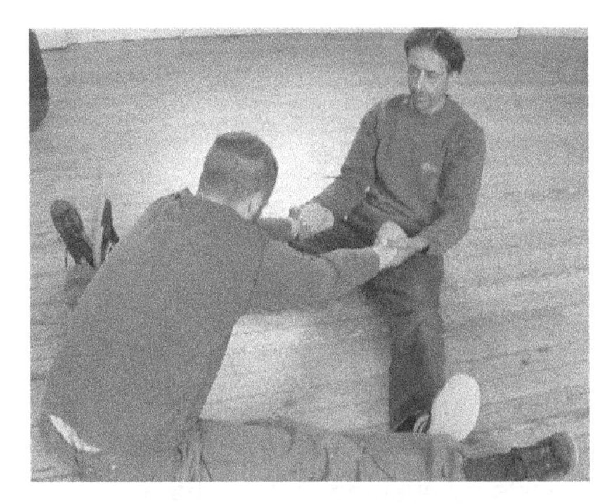

Partners sit facing each other, legs outstretched. PB places his feet inside PA's ankles. Both clasp hands and PB helps PA bend forward, pulling slightly on the hands. PB can also push their feet outwards a little.

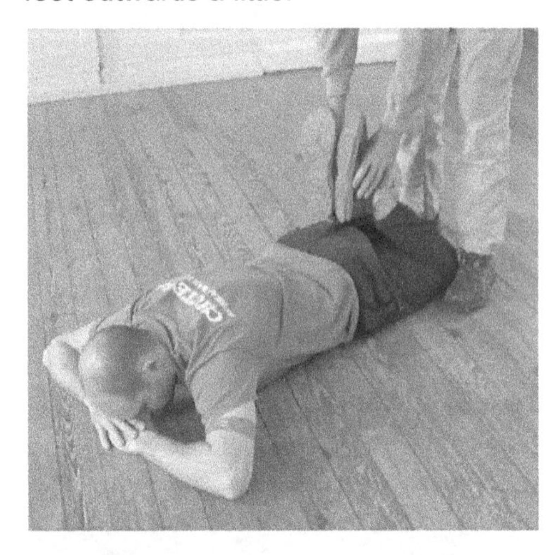

PA lays on their front. PB lifts the feet and slowly moves them towards the backside. Hold the final position for a short time, then release slowly.

PA stands with back to the wall. PB squats and places PA's ankle on their shoulder. PB slowly straightens up, lifting PA's foot. Go slow and pause to breath at each point of tension. PA should keep back and hips against the

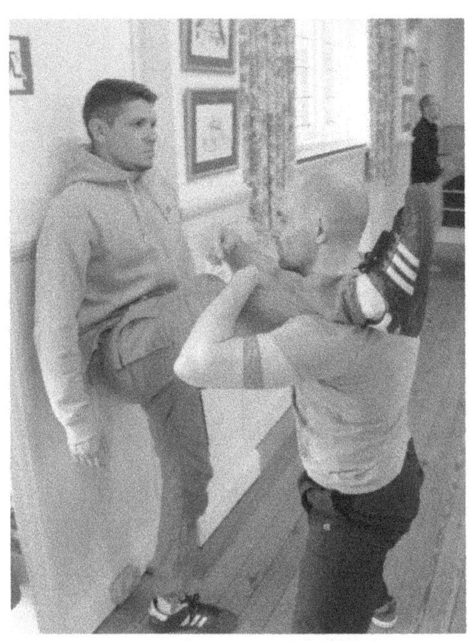

wall. Hold a while at the final position. To finish, PB removes the foot from their shoulder and places the sole of PA's foot onto their own chest. PA now pushes the foot out slowly and allows it to then go to the floor.

PA lays on their back and raises a leg. PB slowly pushes the ankle towards PA's head. Bend the knee and release slowly to finish.

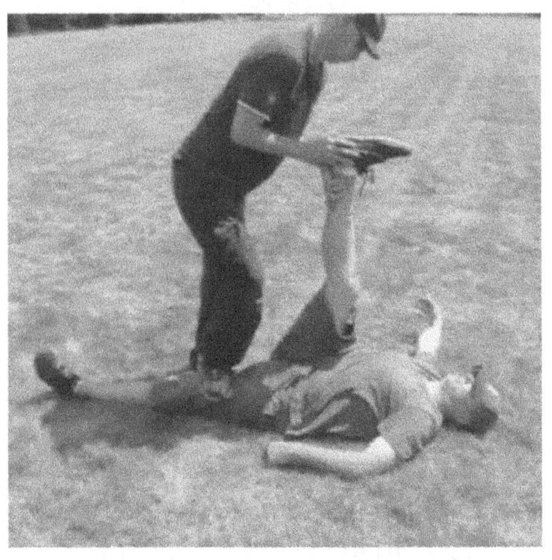

PA lays on their back and raises one knee. PB pushes the knee across to the opposite side. PA can extend the arms out to the sides and should try and keep the shoulders and hips flat on the floor.

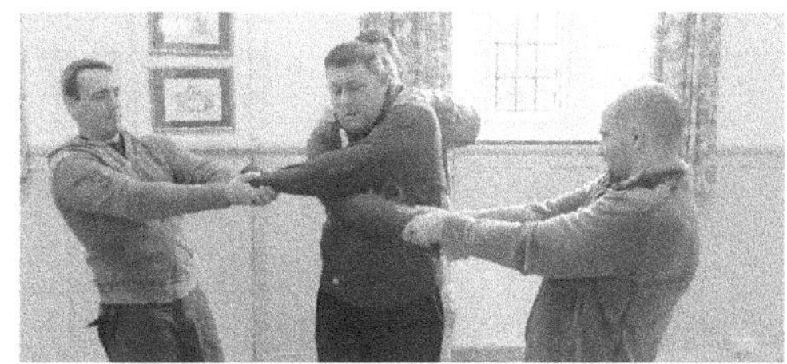

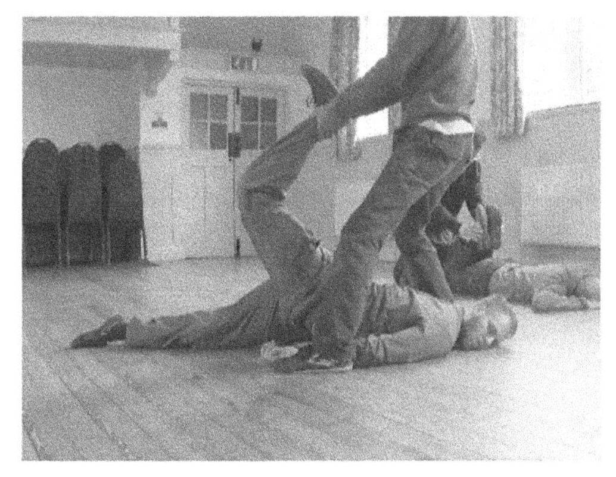

PA lays on their back and raises on foot. PB places the foot on their own chest then slowly leans forward, pushing PA's knee towards their chest. For more random movement, PA lays face up and down on the floor, while PB twists and pulls the legs into as many different positions as possible.

From this I hope you can see that, while there are certainly "fixed" stretching positions, the ultimate aim is to be flexible in all directions. So use the conventional positions as a starting point, then begin to explore as many different movements as you can. You may find it helpful to do some research on anatomy too, good technical knowledge is always useful.

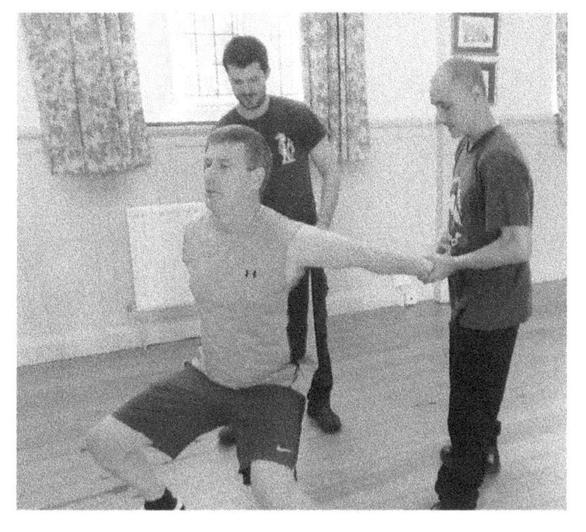

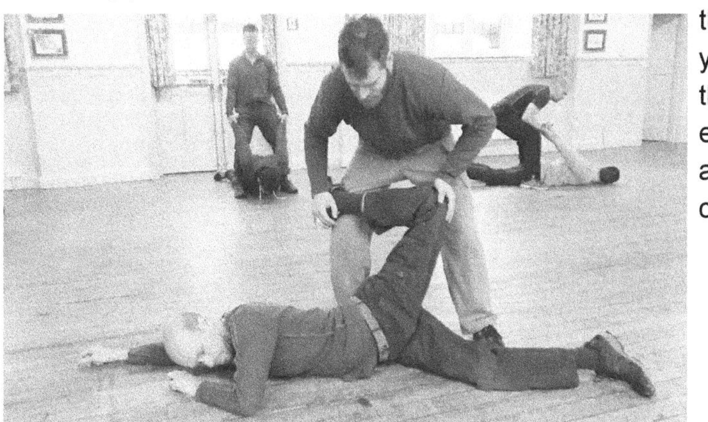

One last thing to mention is that we have shown stretching in pairs but there is nothing to say you can't stretch in threes or more. Just exercise the usual care and caution and be creative!

CHAPTER FIVE
THE HUMAN GYM

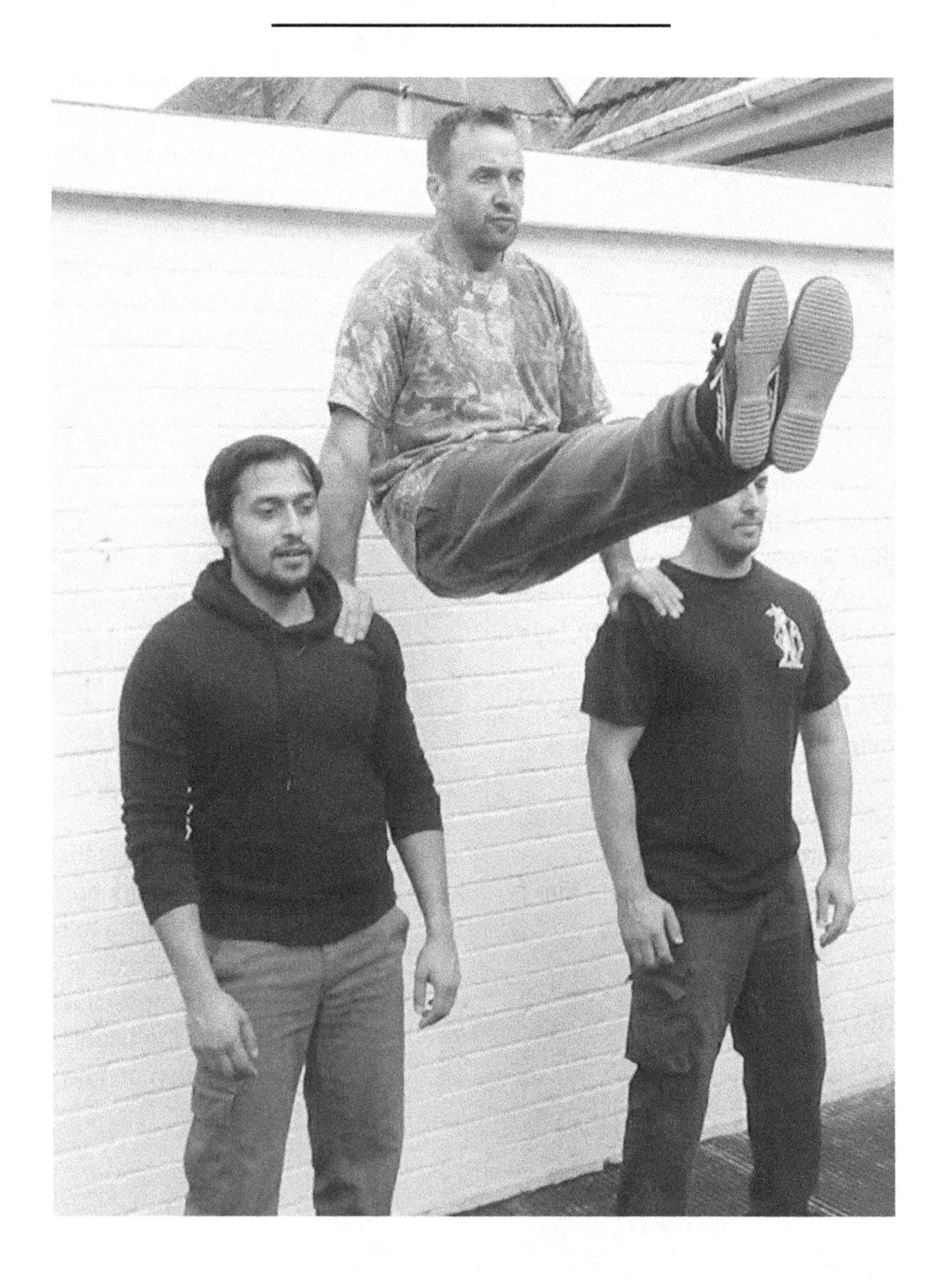

THE HUMAN GYM

When we talk about developing strength, people usually think of gym training, which involves expensive and specialist equipment. How do we train outside of that environment, or when no equipment is available? Simple, we use our training partners!

There are added benefits to this approach. Certain types of gym equipment mean we move and use our muscles in very fixed ways. Everything is very set and stable. People, on the other hand, are decidedly unstable! They are also much more adaptable and sensitive at applying support, resistance and pressure in different planes and directions.

It is also nice to try such training outdoors in the fresh air, I find it gives a different feel to the experience. Training in a group in this way also helps build sensitivity and general group awareness and teamwork.

Many of these exercises build off of the Core Exercises, so it is good to have a good grounding in those before trying some of the more challenging drills. Let's start with some simple work on the hands and arms.

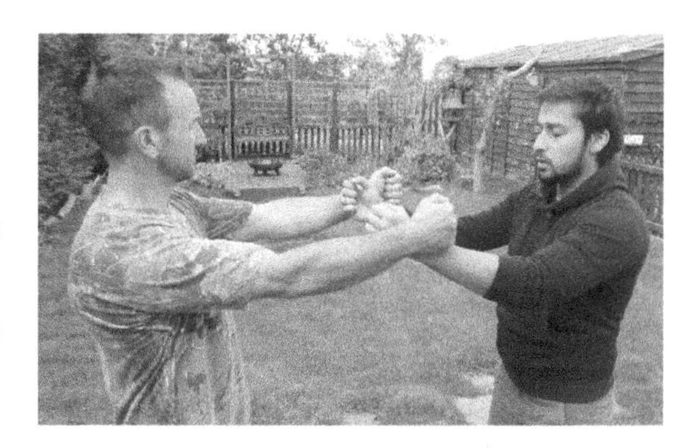

PA extends their arms out at shoulder height. Lock the elbows, close the fists and tense the arms but keep the rest of the body relaxed. PB lays their hands on the fists and builds up gradual downward pressure. When you reach the "bite point" (listen to the breathing!) then maintain a steady pressure. PA tries not to let the fists move at all.

Follow this with upward pressure, inside to out, outside to in, then one hand up, one down, etc. Allow a short break between each change in direction, never change direction suddenly.

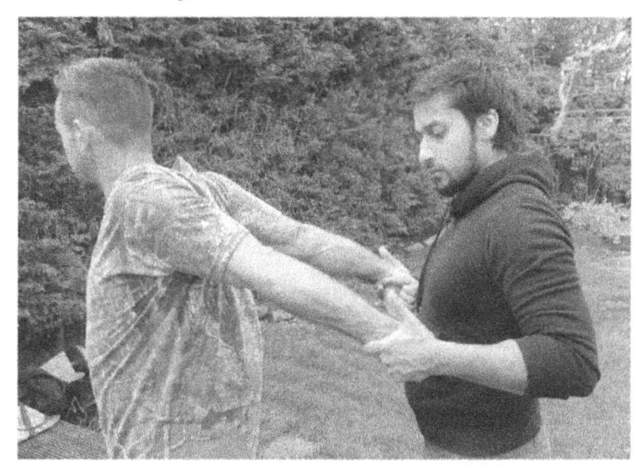

Repeat the same procedure with the hands behind the back. As usual, be aware of tension, posture and breathing. Pay special notice to the legs and hips, don't let them lock up.

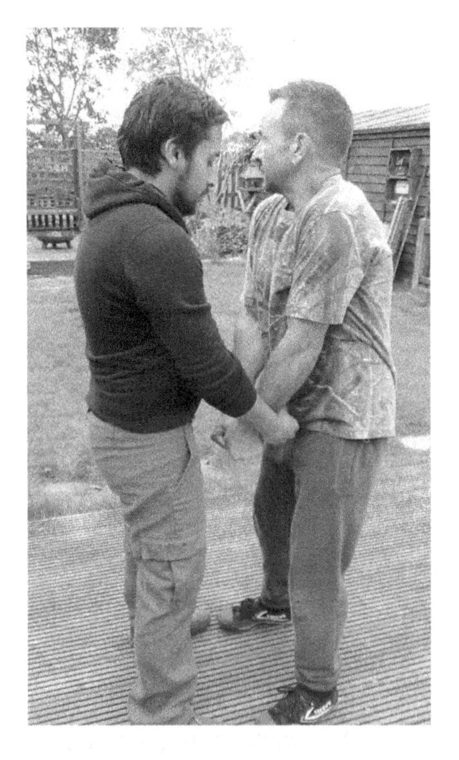

PA and PB face each other, with contact at the wrists. PA's hands are inside, PB's outside. PA lifts their hands above the head. Pause at the top, then PB brings their hands back down to the start position. During each movement, the other partner applies pressure against the

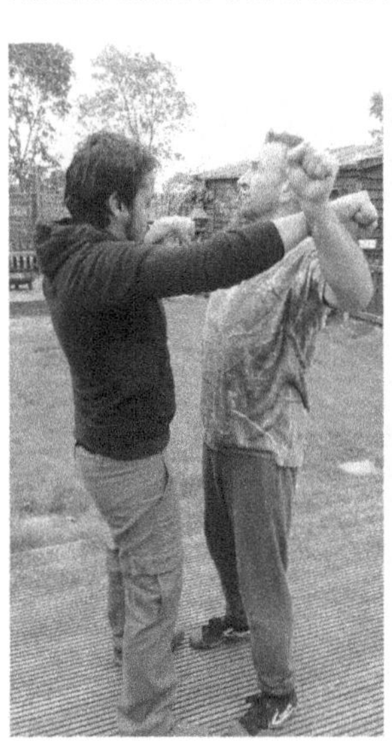

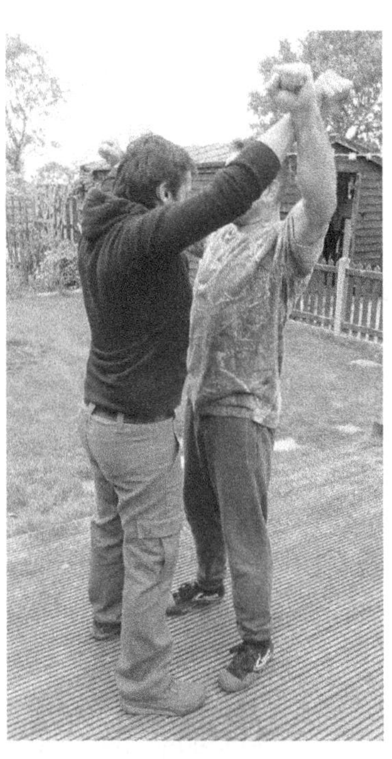

upward or downward movement. This should be gauged.

I suggest at first you run through the move a couple of times with no resistance. Then add a little more resistance each time until it is very difficult for both partners. It should never be impossible though, this is a drill for applying strength through movement!

Pay close attention to the breathing and apply tension only in the arms. The breathing can be a single exhale as you exert or, if working against heavy resistance, a series of burst breaths to help "pump" the arms. Once you have done a certain amount of reps, switch hand positions and repeat.

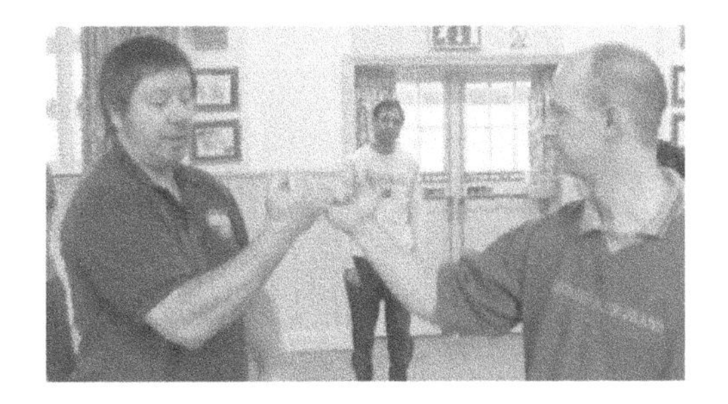

PA AND PB link fingers. Start with the little finger on one hand and work through each of the rest in turn. When linked, both partners apply local tension and pull, matching pressure. Keep the rest of the body relaxed.

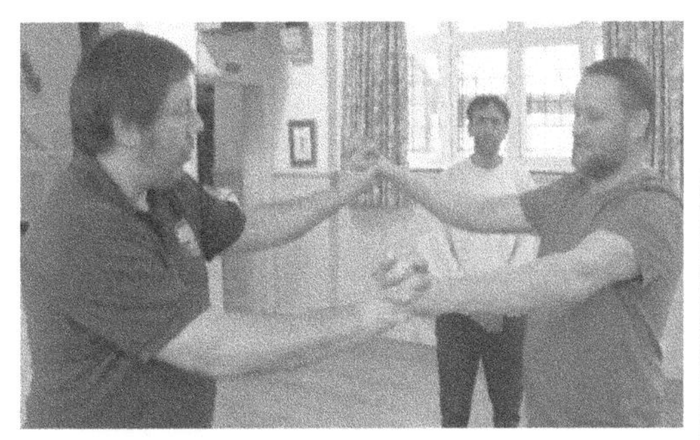

Finish by linking both hands together and slowly pulling and pushing in different directions.

Let's now take a look at a sequence for the legs. PA lays on the floor and raises their feet about six inches. PB stands with legs on the outside of PA's feet. PA now slowly

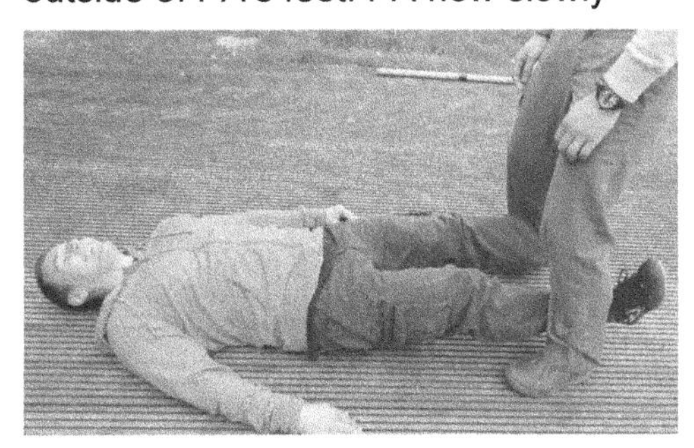

pushes outward, with local tension. PB provides resistance.

Following this, PB switches to the inside position and repeats.

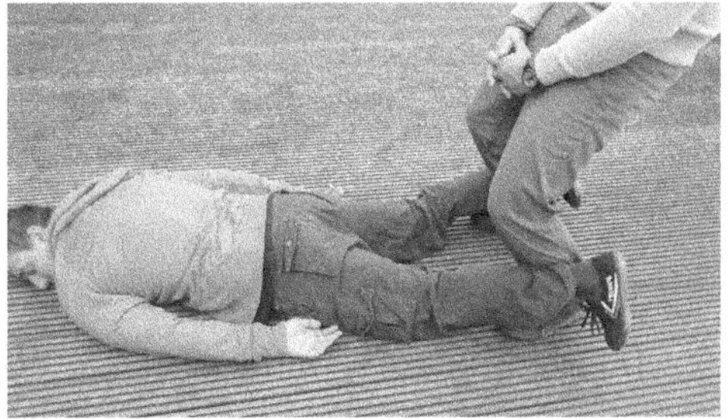

After that, PB places their foot on PA's shin (keep the heel on the ground) and provides resistant as PA tries to lift the leg. Following these,

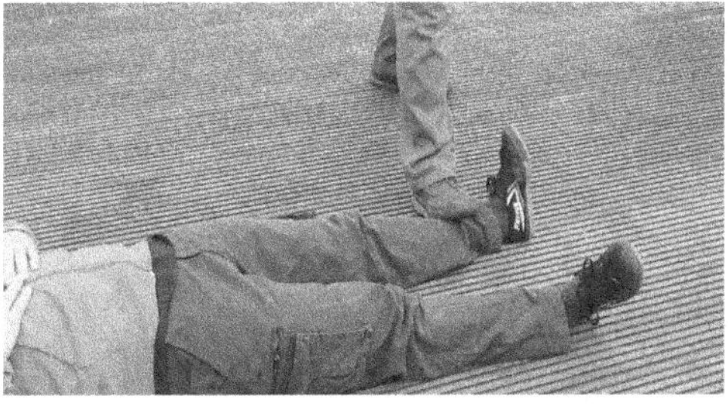

repeat the same procedure with PA laying on their front.

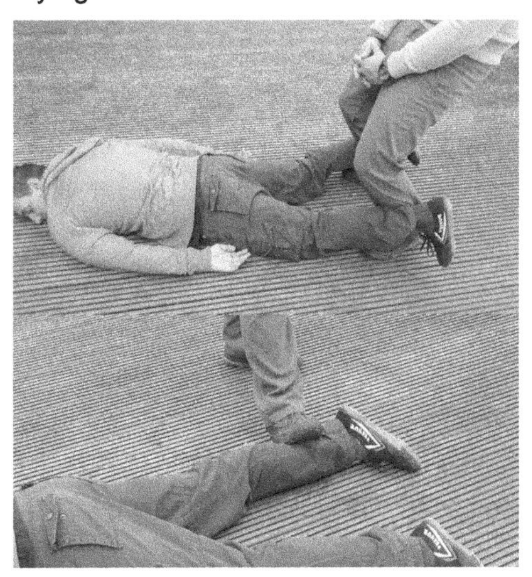

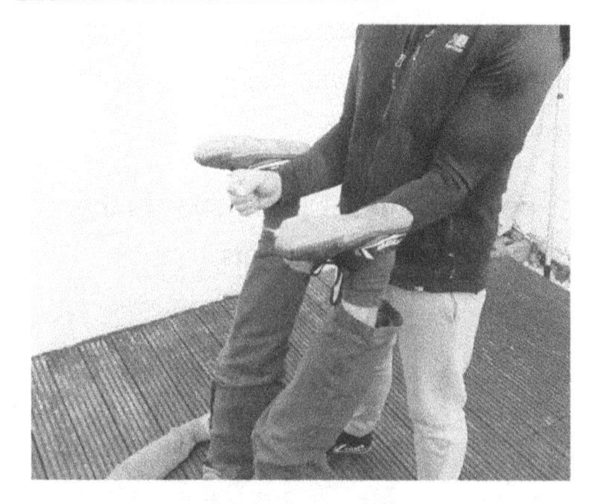

You can work in a similar way by resisting with the arms rather than the legs. In this case PA raises their legs to 90 degrees. From this position you can move the feet inwards, outwards and also back and forwards against resistance.

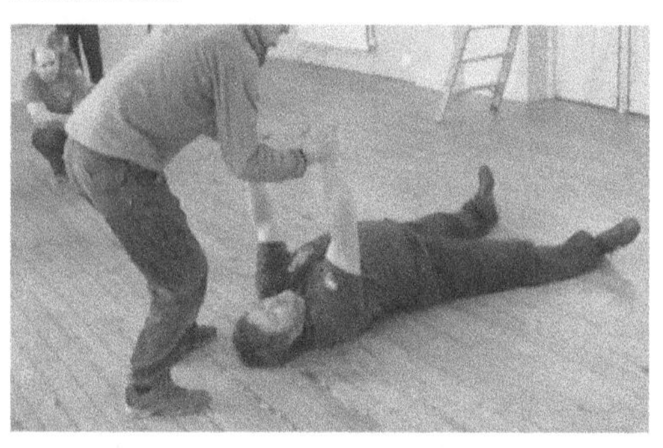

You can also work the same method against the raised arms. Keep the arms straight and work against resistance in all directions. Once more, keep the rest of the body relaxed.

It may seem on many exercises that only one person is getting to do the work, the other is just providing support or resistance. However we can use the idea of resistance to give both partners a workout at the same time. For example, to work the legs, partners press the knees against each other. Apply gradual, matching pressure with local tension. After a while, change angle and position. Take care of the knees!

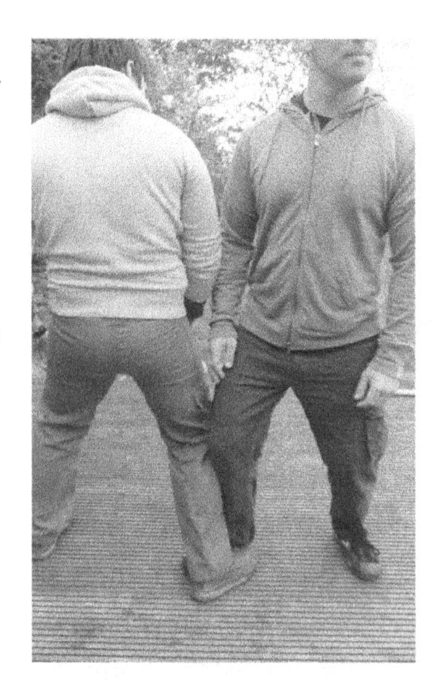

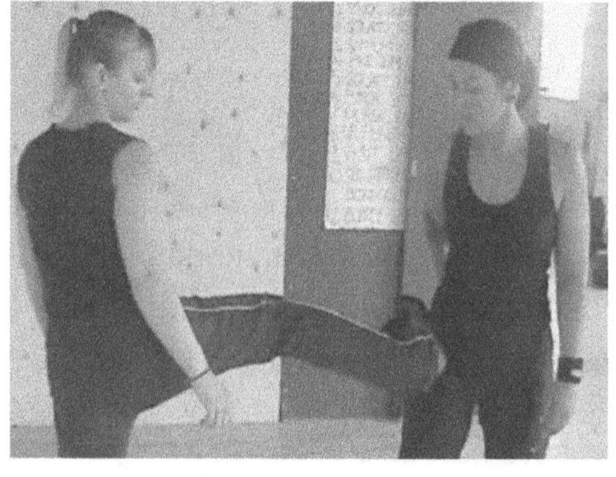

We can work the idea of resistance in order to develop our kicks too. Begin in a static position, with PA placing their foot against PB's body and slowly pushing out. PB can vary the level of resistance. Once again work as many different angles and positions as you can. PA should make sure they are keeping an upright posture and are not leaning into the push.

You can then make this into a moving exercise. This time PA places the foot and pushes PB back, then immediately steps forward and repeats with the other foot. Keep the

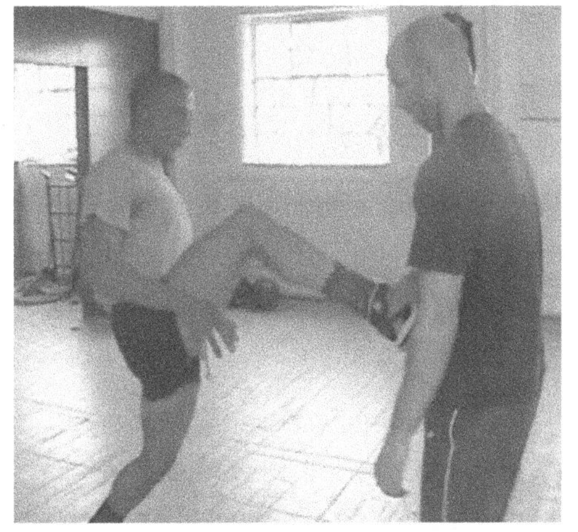

movement fluid and once again ensure the body remains upright. PB can vary the amount of resistance. Work from one end of the room to the other, then switch roles and return.

The next exercise can be a challenge and so should be approached carefully and gradually. PA kneels (sun hat optional) and PB holds down the ankles. PA now slowly leans forward, keeping the back

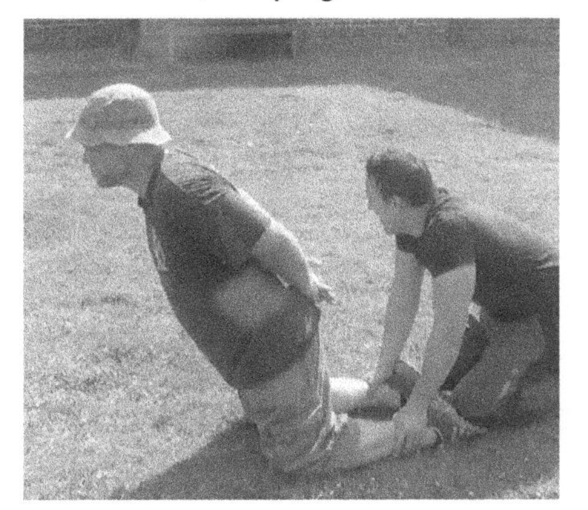

straight. Please do not go too far forward the first time you try this! Going forward is easy, coming back is more difficult!

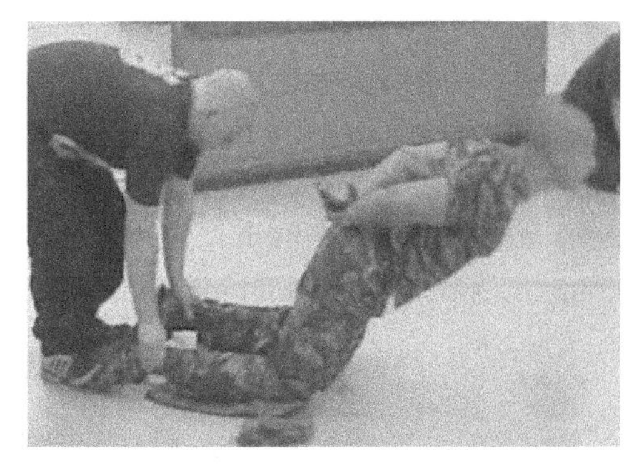

Work a small lean, then gradually build up. Make sure you keep good form. With practice you will be able to lean further forward before returning to the start position. It is even possible to "kiss the floor" with this movement.

Having done some work on the legs, let's return to the arms. PA faces PB and places their fist on PB's chest. PA stands in a forward stance and PB slowly leans forward, lifting the heels.

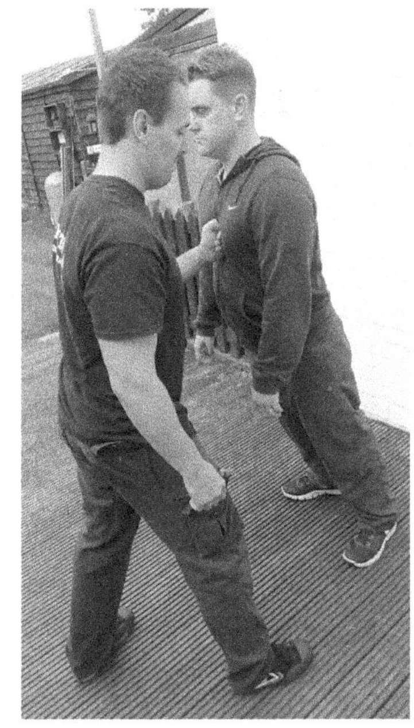

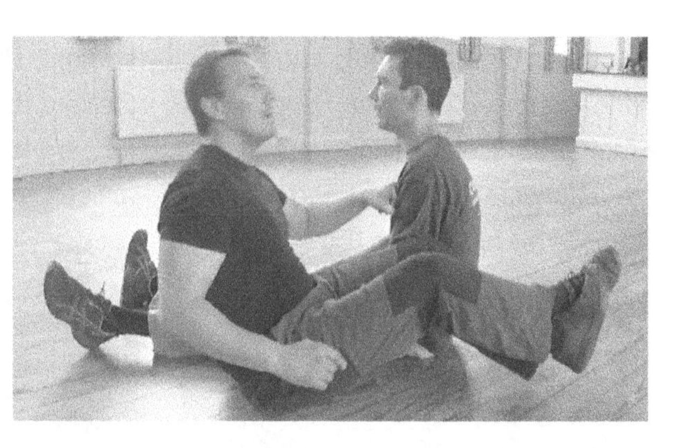

PA inhales and takes PB's full weight onto the fist, allowing it to come back, sinking a little into the rear leg. Once the fist is in line with the body, PA exhales, pushes up from the back foot and pushes the fist out, so moving PB backwards. The movement should be smooth and with minimal tension. Think of the back leg as a spring, which is loaded then released.

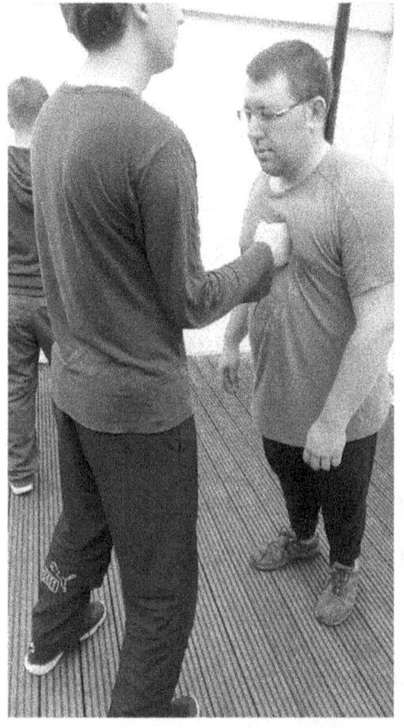

Once you can do this easily, try the next step. Instead of a forward stance, PA stands in a more normal position. Now there is less reliance on the back leg. See how you can generate movement from the hip instead.

Following this, A stands with feet parallel. Now you have to find a point of support from which to push the fist out. Remember, the legs should stay relaxed and not locked. Push the fist out without "grounding". You can try using shoulder rotation at first, after a time you will learn to develop points of support within the body from which you can send out a strike.

As variations, you can try on one leg, sitting down with feet raised, or on a slippery surface. The aim is to learn how to deliver a punch without relying on stance. You can follow the same routine and apply the push via a shoulder, elbow, knee or kick. Once again try and work from that "floating root" principle. Don't just push forward either, work sideways, back, down ,etc.

For the next exercise we adopt a "sticky hands" position. Partners contact at the wrists and begin to

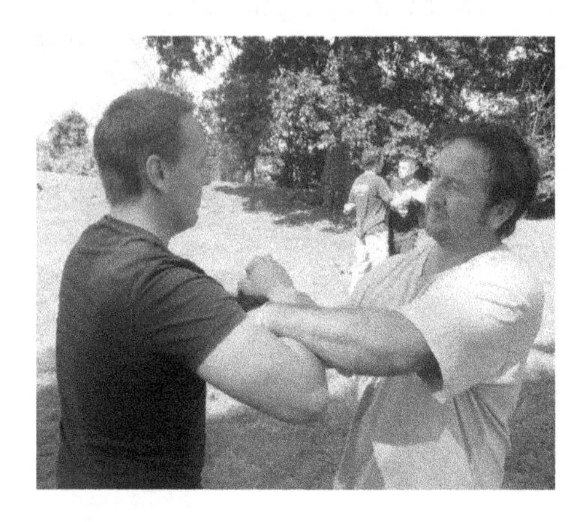

slowly move the arms, maintaining an even pressure. Now begin to build up the local tension, resisting each other but still moving slowly. Take care not to

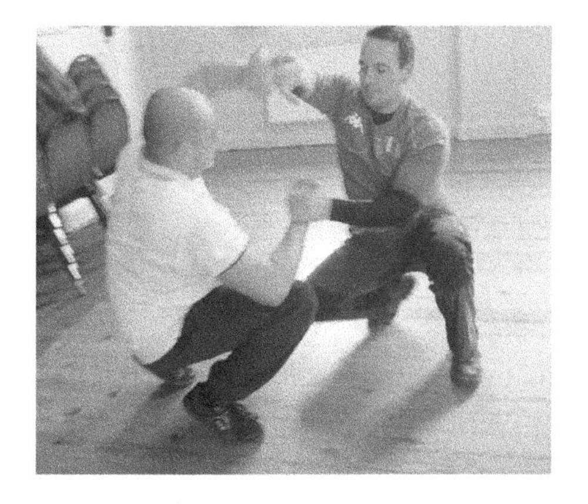

lock the shoulders, hips or legs.

For variation, change level as you do the exercise, until you are working from a squat position. You can also try working in groups of three or more. Remember, the aim is to maintain even contact and pressure throughout.

Another selective tension exercise is to have your partner push on one part of the body. Your job is to tense just that particular spot and not let it be moved. Pushes start with one hand and then progress to two. So your partner may

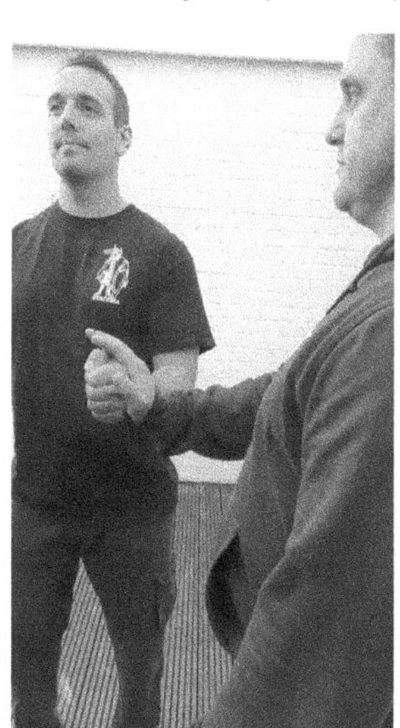

push on your forehead and hip at the same time. Try and connect the two points of contact with a single line of tension. Breathe and maintain posture.

The converse of this exercise is to totally relax as you are pushed and we will describe this later. However here is an interesting mix of tension and relaxation in one drill! You need three people, so time to say hello to Partner C!

PA stands with arms held out in front. PB and PC take an arm each. Both then slowly move each arm around. PA's job is to allow one arm to

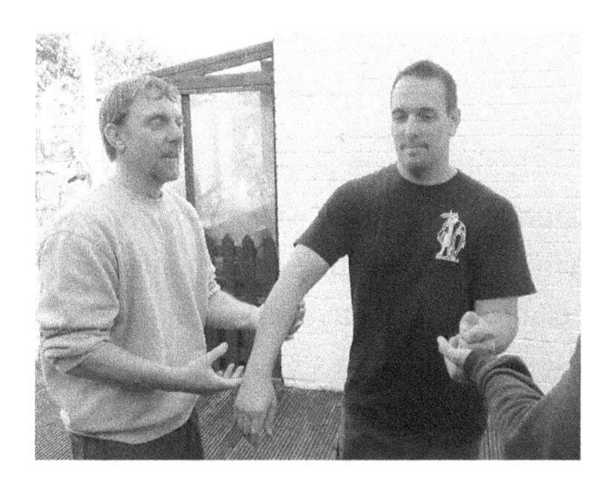

be moved freely but to keep the other locked firmly in place. This is quite a challenge so take it slow. There are considerable benefits to be gained from this kind of work, the ability to selectively control individual muscle groups has a host of applications.

Once you have worked the arms you can, of course, also try the same method with the legs.

WORKING IN THREES

As we have now introduced PC, let's look at some trio exercises. Two people can give one a lot of support, so we will start with some "assisting" drills.

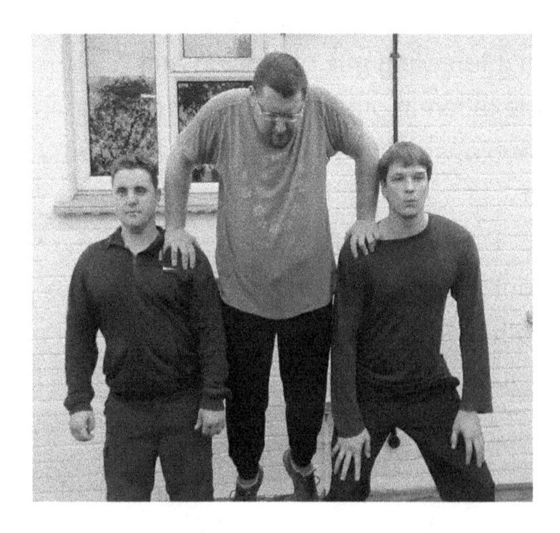

PB and PC stand side by side. PA supports themselves with a hand on each partner's shoulder. From this position PA can practice dips and leg raises.

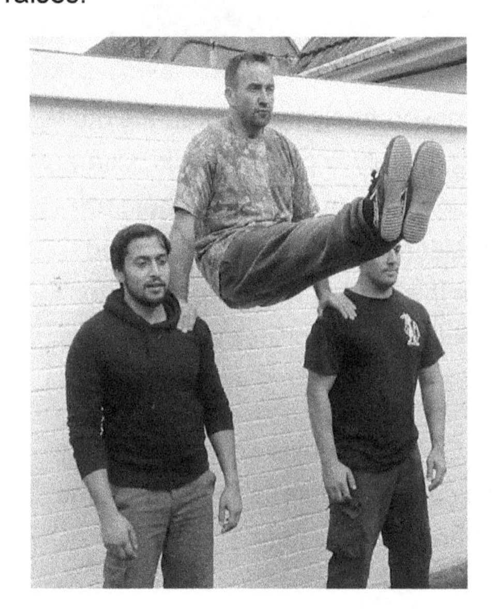

At first the supporting partners should stay still. However, as a progression they can beginning to squat or move around slightly in order to make the support less solid.

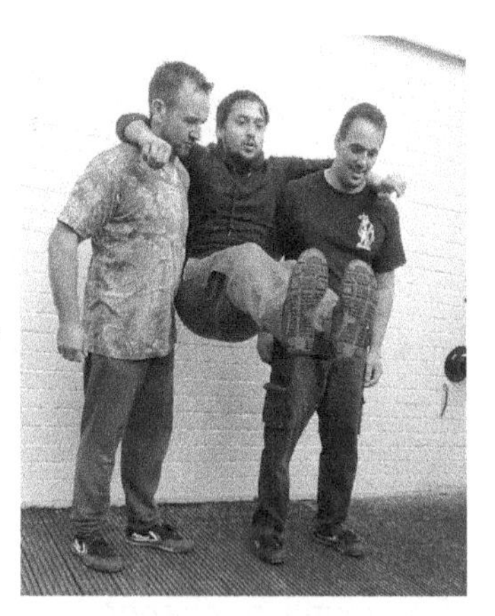

For a leg raise variation, PA drapes arms over the support er's shoulder. This gives more of a solid base to work from so is a good place to start from.

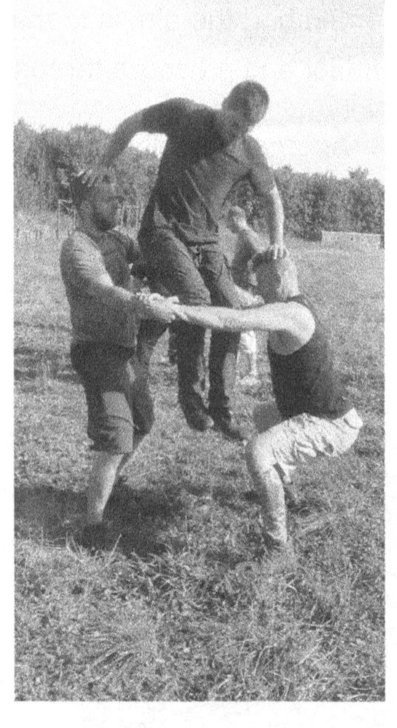

You don't have to use the shoulders for support. PB and PC can link arms and PA can use the heads as support. Be sure the no-one involved has neck problems. The support partners can be static or move as before.

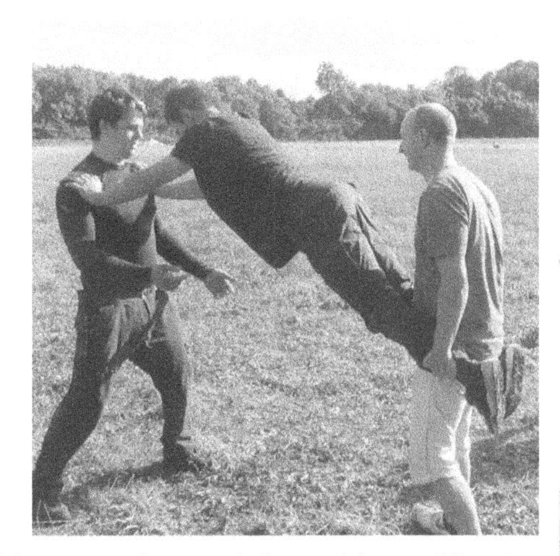

You can also work from this position to use your supporters as a climbing frame. See if you can climb up and onto their shoulders. Alternatively have PB hold your ankles while you "climb" up and down PC's body. You need robust clothing for this one!

If we add a stick into the mix we get another range of exercises. Make sure the sticks will support your weight!

PB and PC support the stick on their shoulders while PA does pull ups. There are lots of variations from this basic position. Rather than pull ups, PA can hang and do leg raises. These can be out to 90 degrees or higher. You can easily turn this into a pull up and over the stick.

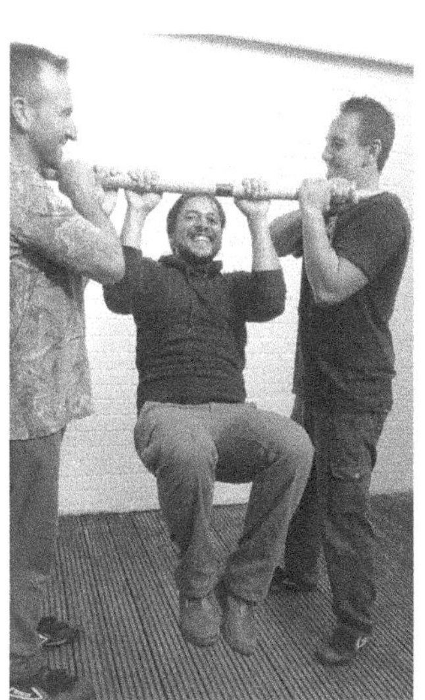

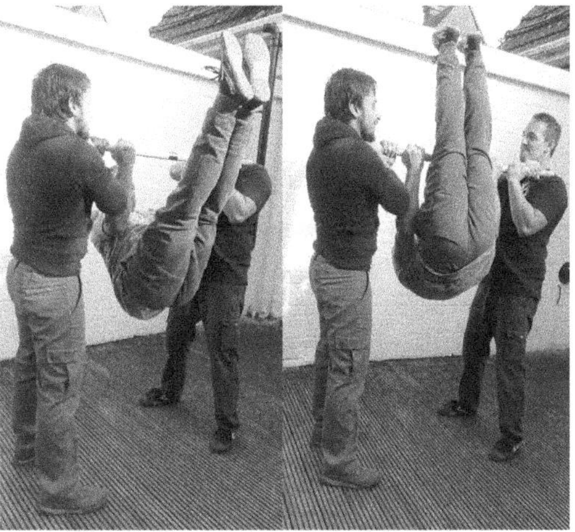

For more basic variations, try changing your grip, working with one arm, or working dips rather than pulls. You can even try hanging from your feet and lifting the body!

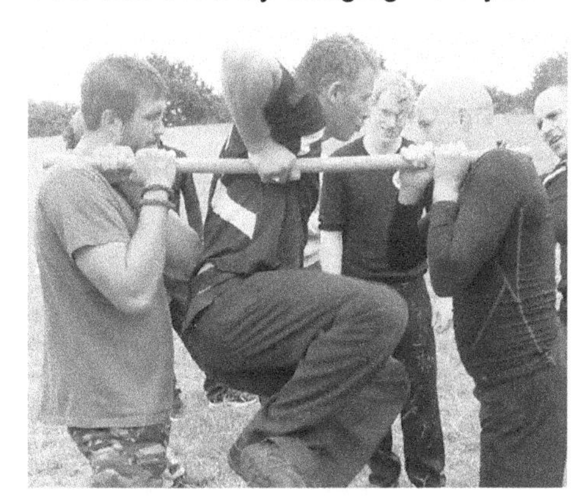

FOURS AND MORE

If two people can give us a lot of support, imagine how much we can get from four! We can take most of the pair exercises and convert them into a group of four but there are also plenty of additional drills we can work with a group.

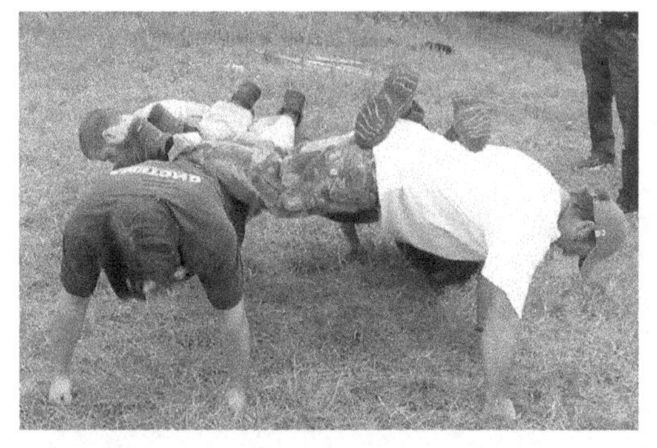

The square push up is an example. The four partners get in push up position, with feet placed on the upper back of the person behind them. The aim is to work synchronised movement and breathing, so lower and raise as one unit.

For the aerial push up, PA rests feet and hands on four supporters and

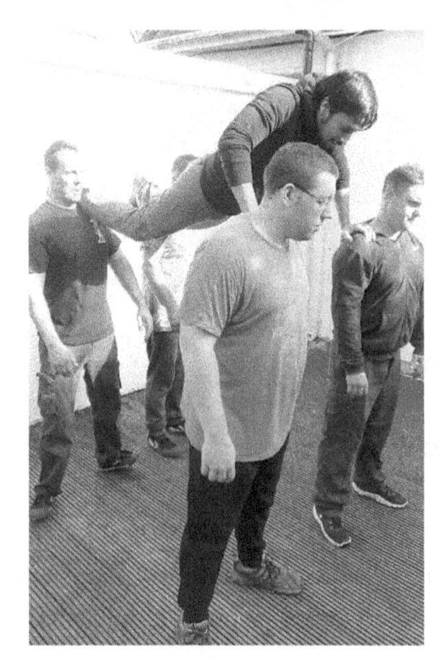

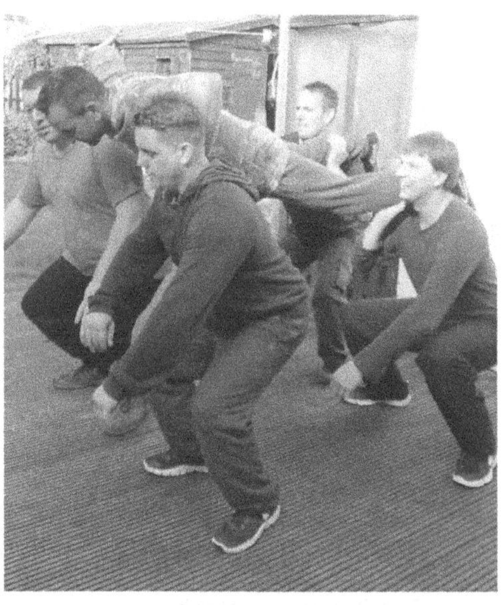

performs push ups. For the first level, the supporters should be static.

Once you can do this, the supporters can beginning squatting, either in unison or individually. For a further challenge, rather than rest on the shoulders, rest on the supporters' hands.

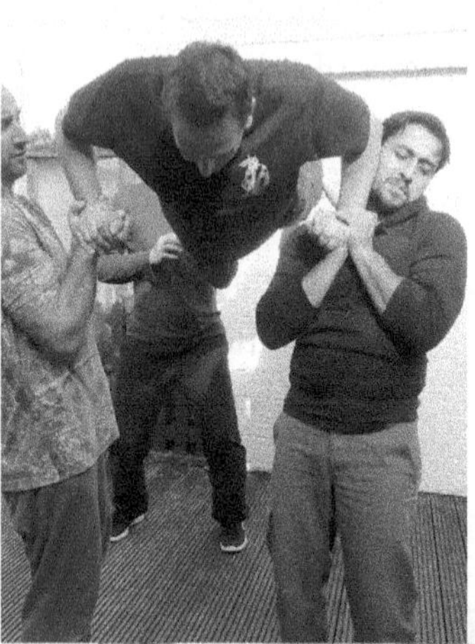

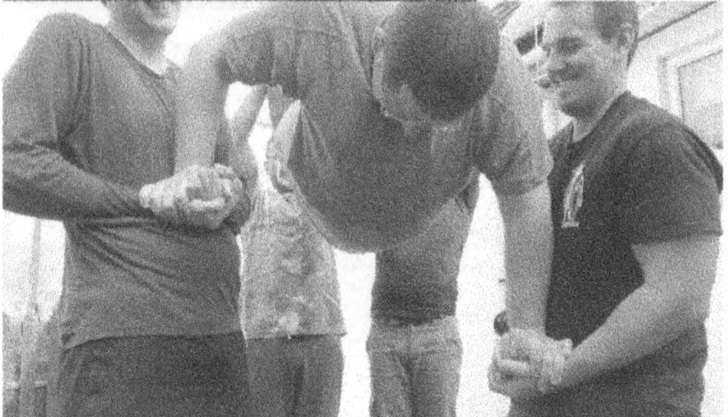

You can add a further level of challenge into this by then having the supporters raise / move their hands around too.

We can work a similar idea with the sticks. This time one pair holds a stick under the feet, the other holds a stick under

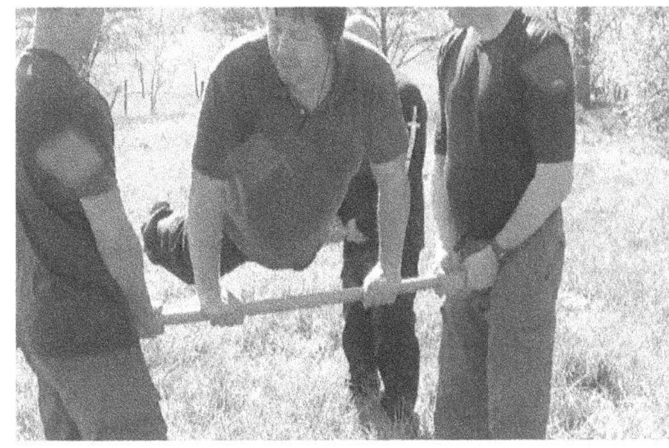

As before, move the sticks in order to increase the challenge.

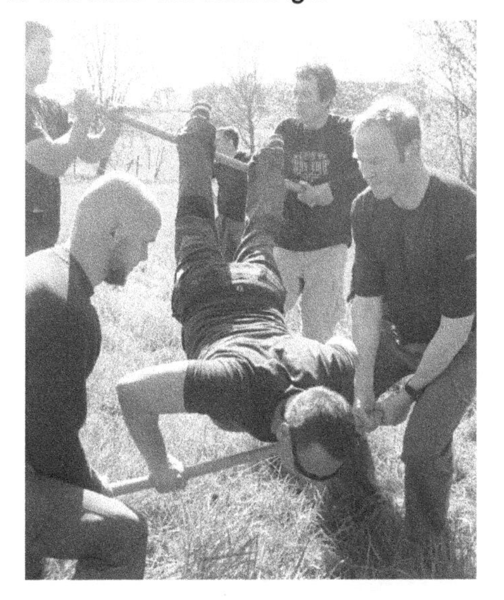

Another group push up variation is for the group to get into a circle, facing

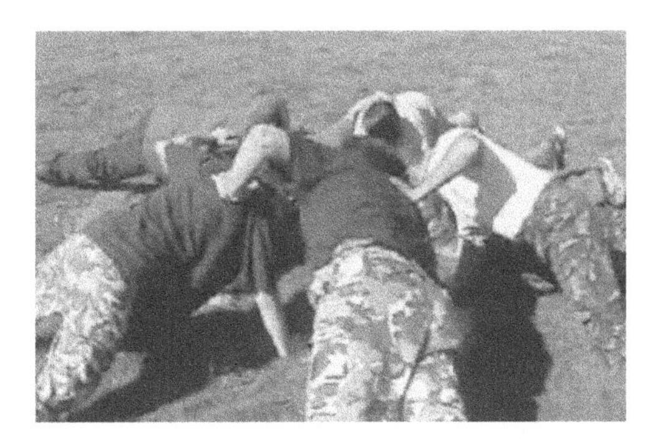

inwards, in push up position. Each person then places their left hand on the shoulder of the person to their left. The right hand remains on the floor. At the signal, the group synchronises push ups. After your set or repetitions, repeat with the other hand down.

Other possibilities with pairs or groups include carry drills. Pairs simply have to carry each other over a certain distance. Let people experiment with different ways to pick up and carry. You can make any of these drills a race between groups if you wish.

You can also run this as a team exercise if you have enough people.

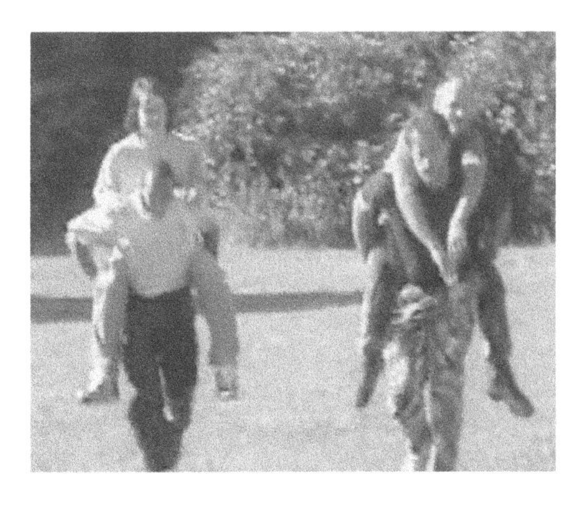

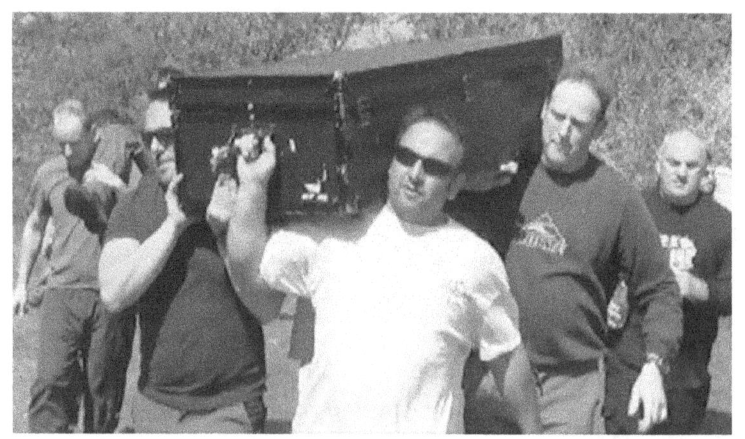

Split into groups of four of five and designate a course, or follow a leader. The group have to jog the course whilst carrying one of the members. The member should be switched around from time to time. You could also substitute use a bulky object, add in obstacles and/or place restrictions on the teams.

Larger groups are also good for climbing exercises. The group stands close together while on or more persons climbs up to stand on the shoulders.

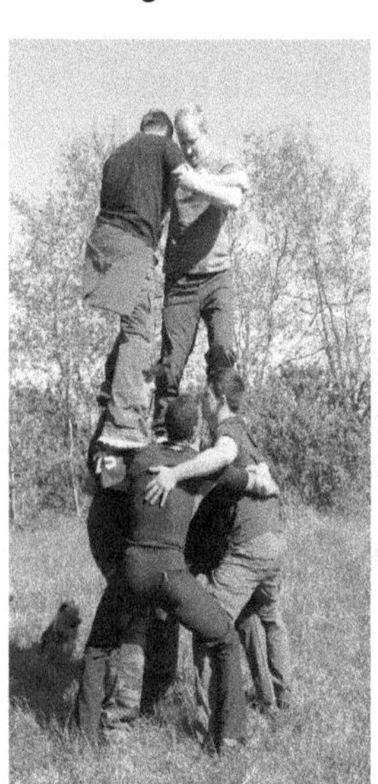

There are also gauntlet type exercises we can run with a large group. Check everyone is ok with the next one before trying! The group lay face up in a line and take it in turns to walk along the line, stepping on everyone's stomach. We suggest going slow at first and be mindful of where you place your feet! Later on you can speed up if you wish.

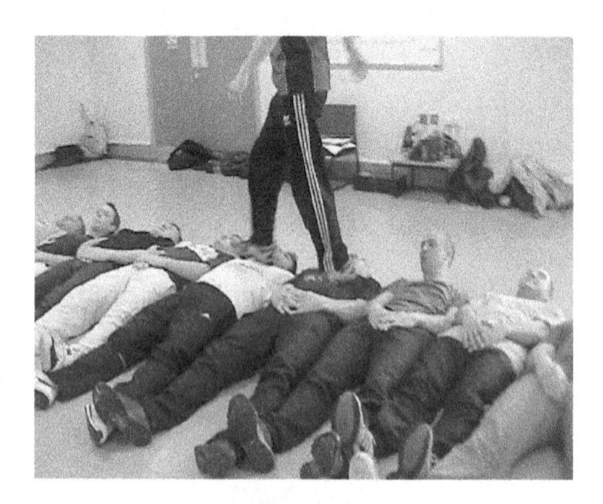

Along similar lines, have the group rotate and get into push up position. Again, in turn from the end, one person has to crawl quickly under the whole group.

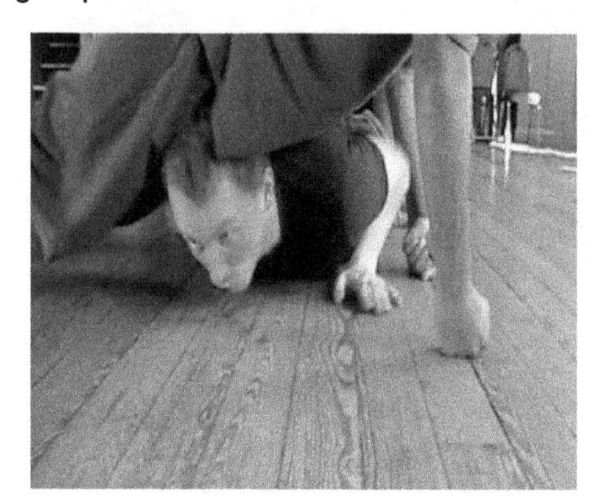

For a good leg workout, get the whole group into a circle, with arms around the shoulders. The group goes into squat position. At the signal, the group begins to hop, either to the left or to the right. Synchronise breathing and movement! Pause, then go back the other way.

To finish this section, let's go back to some partners drills, based around the idea of support. Simply lifting a partner is an easy one, but find different and new ways to do it!

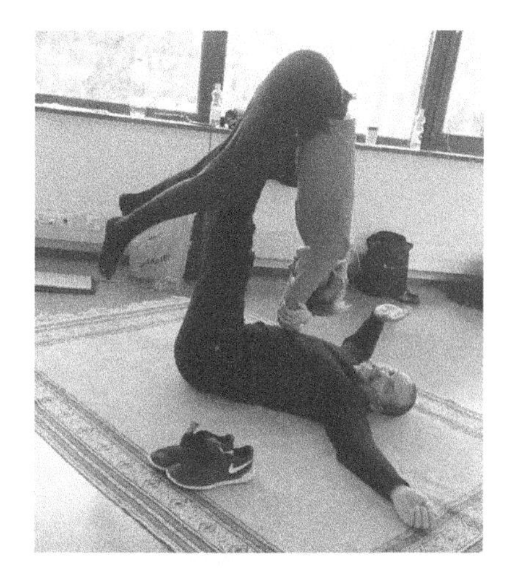

Challenge each other to come up with different variations on the core exercises. There are a ton of ideas,

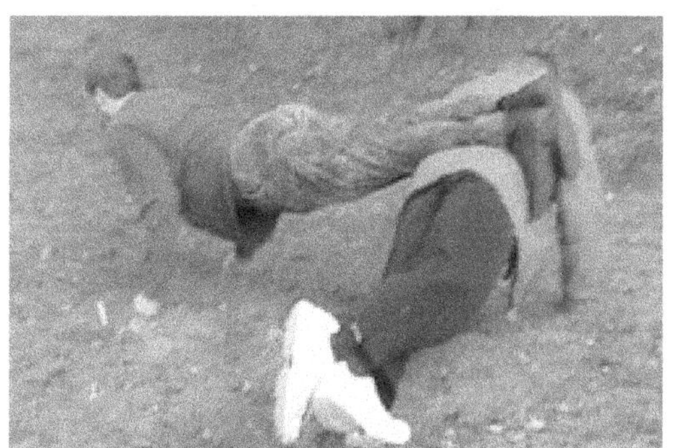

with push ups, for example two of you can try a "half square", or the one handed push up.

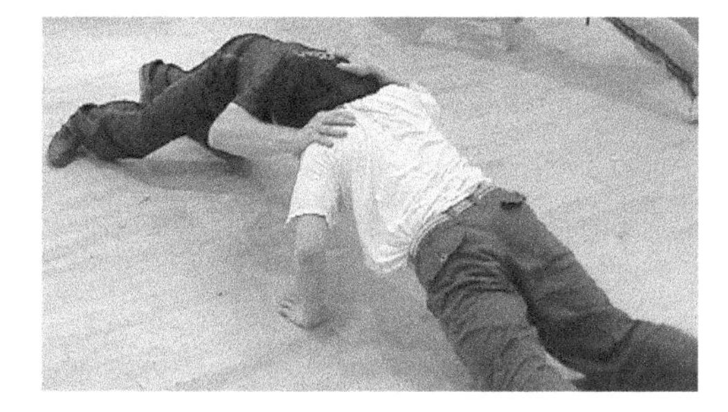

You can even try doing push ups on push ups!

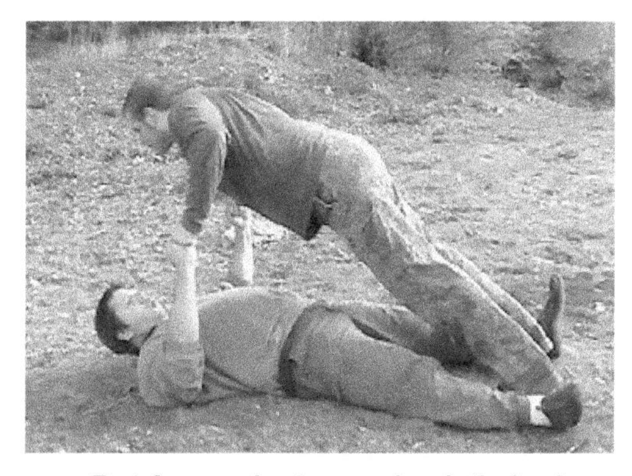

But for our last exercise let's look at a body tension drill. This is a little challenging, be sure there are no neck issues before you start. PA and PB stand face to face, each places a hand on the others forehead. At the signal, each slowly shuffles their feet back, keeping the body straight and strong. Enjoy!

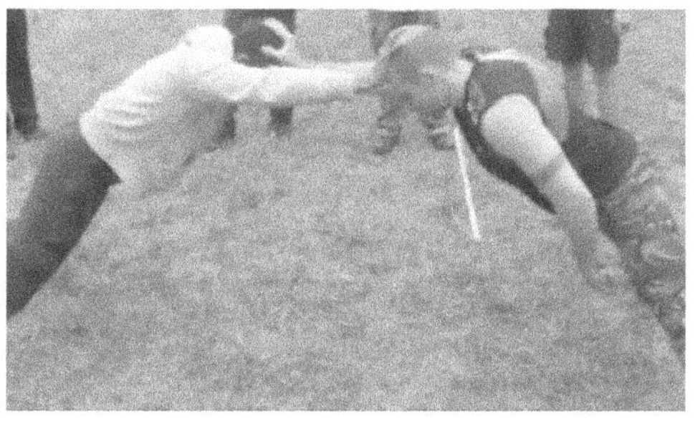

CHAPTER SIX
PADWORK

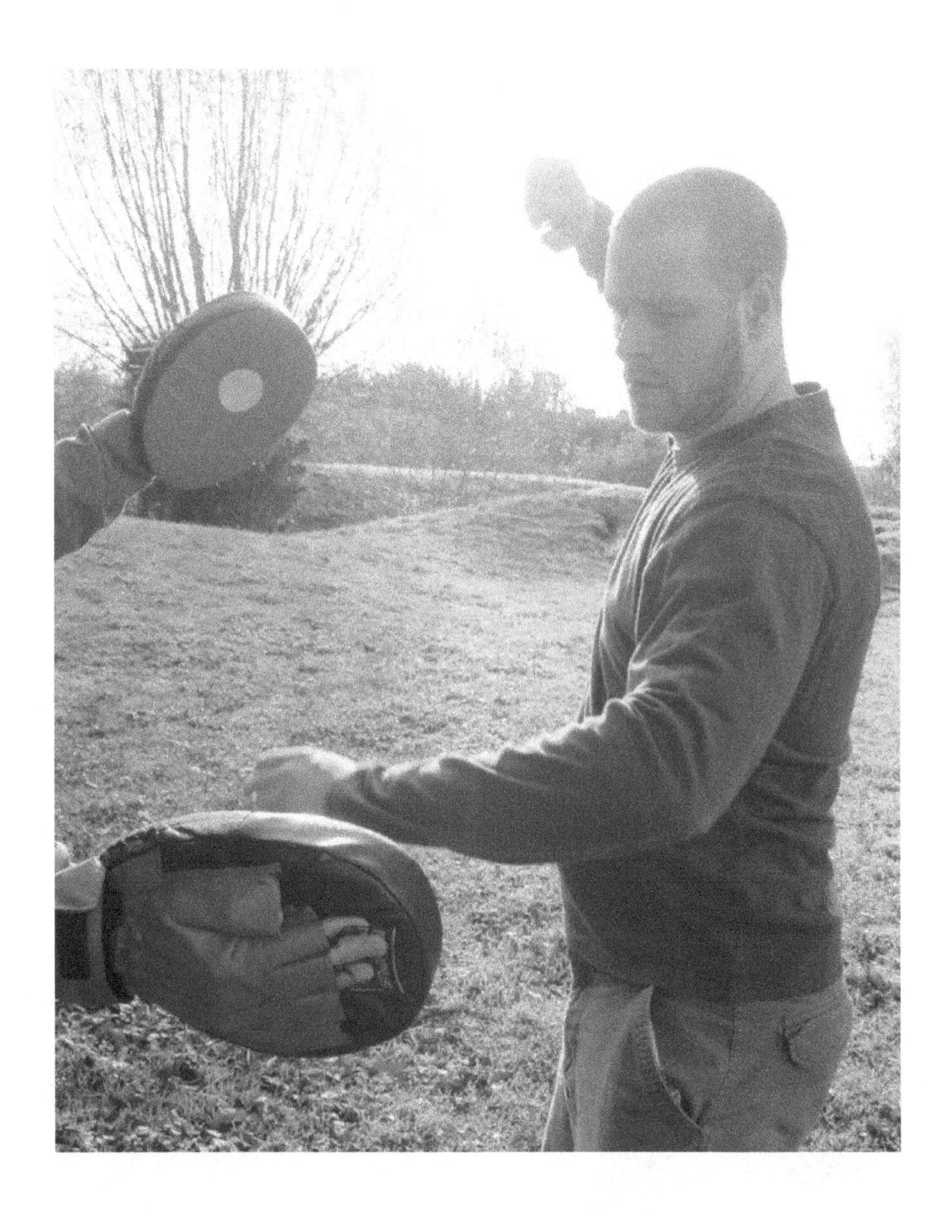

PADWORK

Focus pads are a great piece of partner training kit, however we should be aware that pads have pros and cons. On the plus side, they are good for developing speed, combinations of strikes and, of course, we can hit them at full power. On the downside they can lead to unrealistic distancing / targeting and there is also the "pad effect" - this is when people see a pad and feel they have to hit it as hard as they can, to the detriment of form, relaxation and awareness.

Be aware of these issues in any pad work and you will be fine. A lot also depends on the pad holder. For example, I have seen people hold the

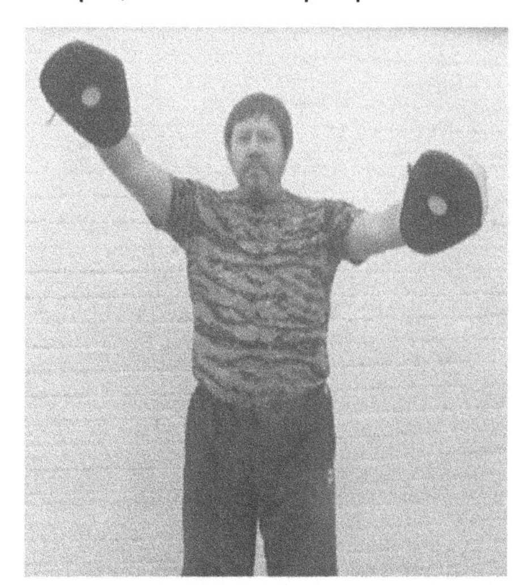

pads like so. This may be due to nerves, or just not knowing how to position the pads properly.

First let's look at the angle of the pad. People typically hold them at 90 degrees to start, which creates two problems. First, It is difficult to absorb the impact of the strike so will be uncomfortable for the wrists. Second, there are very few targets which are at a 90 degree angle, unless you are punching a wall.

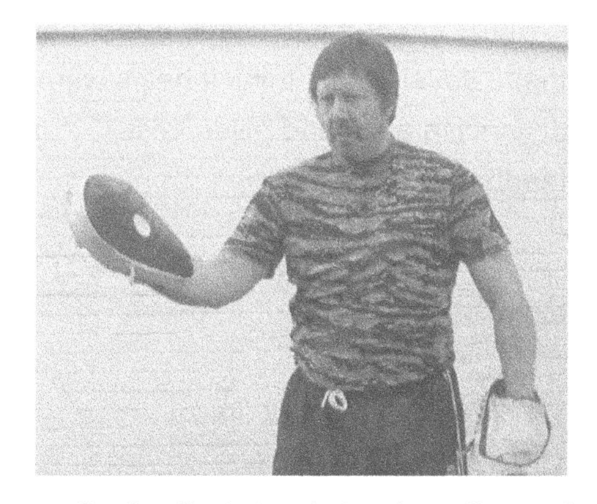

So the first step is to place the pad at an angle that matches the target area of the strike. If this is a downward blow to the chest, for example, hold the pad at a slight angle at chest height.

For the most part I prefer to hold the pads close to the body. This helps

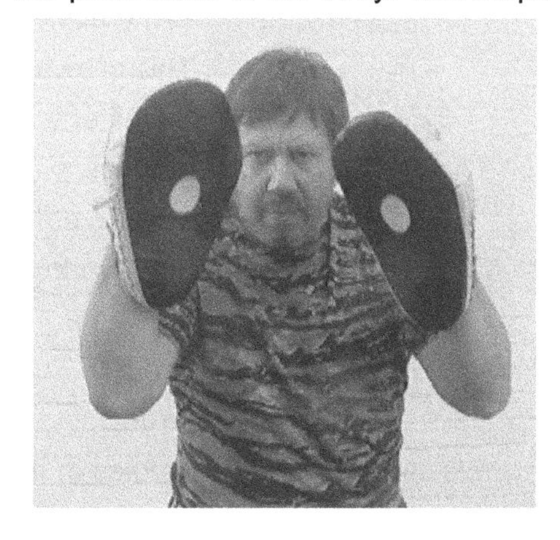

the holder absorb impact but also gets you used to being close to strikes. So if you are practicing face punches (and you trust your partner!) hold the pads close to your face. I like to hold the hands quite firm, with just a bit of give. Enough to protect the pad holders joints, but not to be too soft a target. I don't agree with pushing the pad towards the strike as some trainers do these days. I don't think it helps with distancing at all and gives false feedback.

So let's look at some specific exercises.

STATIC DRILLS

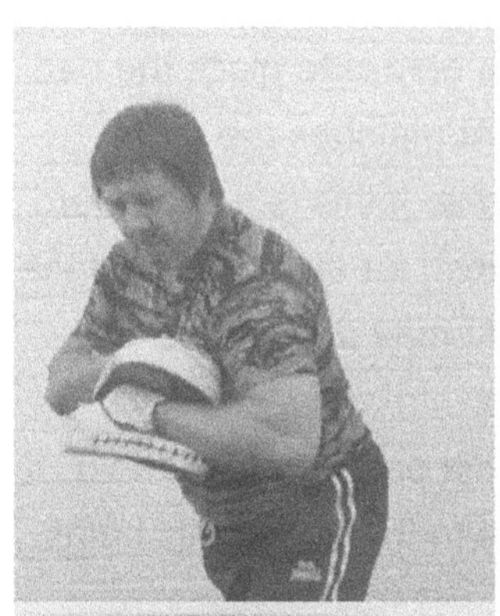

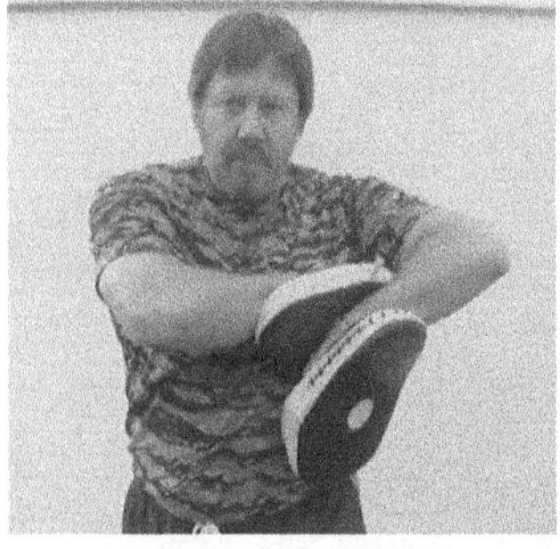

These are where the pad holder remains on the spot and generally keeps the pads in the same place. This allows the hitter to practice a specific strike or to work against a specific target.

We can see a few examples in the

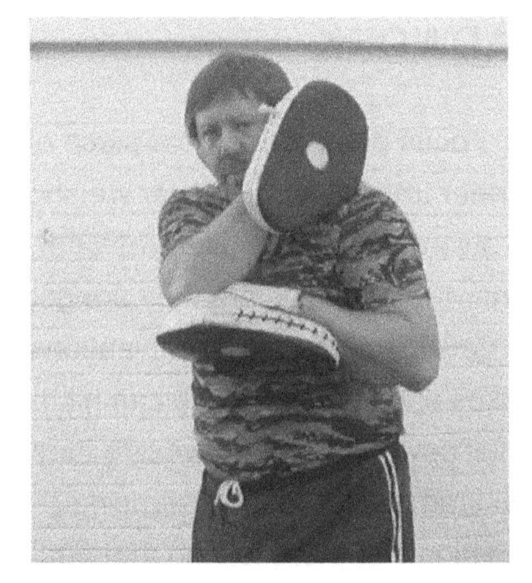

photos, for working body shots, knees strikes and so on.

BASIC STRIKES

Hold the pads at shoulder height. The hitter practices hooks, jabs and/or Figure Eight strikes. Start slow and work on good posture, movement and breathing to start.

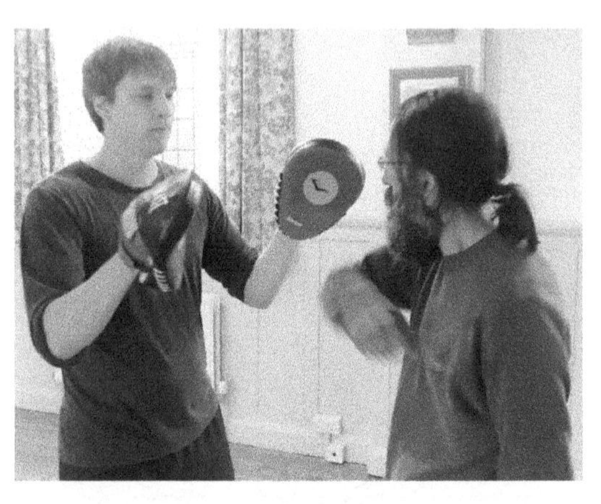

Work the same method with punches to the body and also elbows and knees

From here you can begin to increase speed. Try to develop a flow

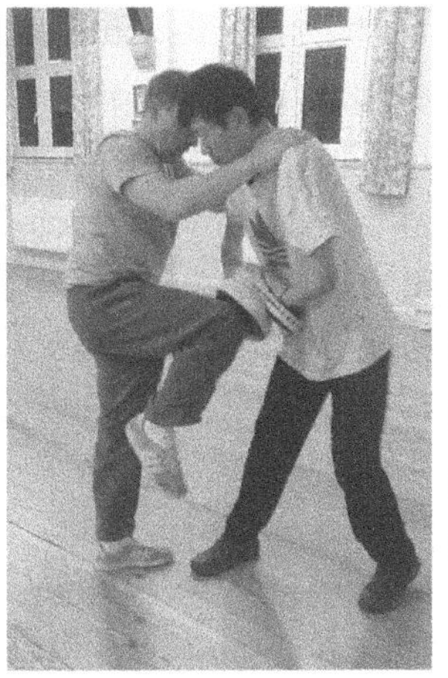

and keep your movements smooth. A good workout is to do any of the above for a set time at maximum speed.

A simple variation on the basic drills is to add

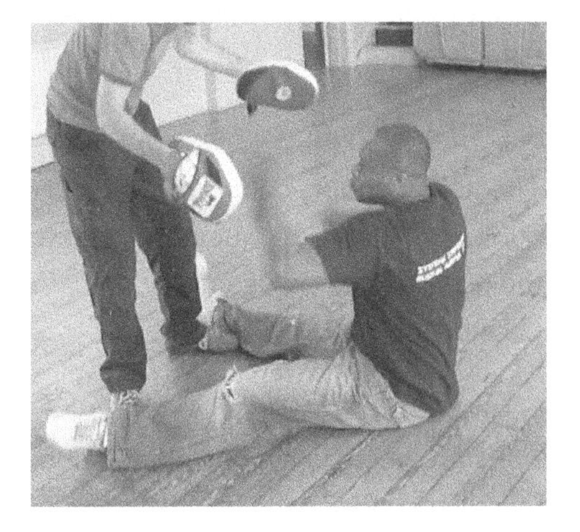

some form of restriction in for the hitter. They may be sitting in a chair, able to use only one arm, be prone on the floor, etc.

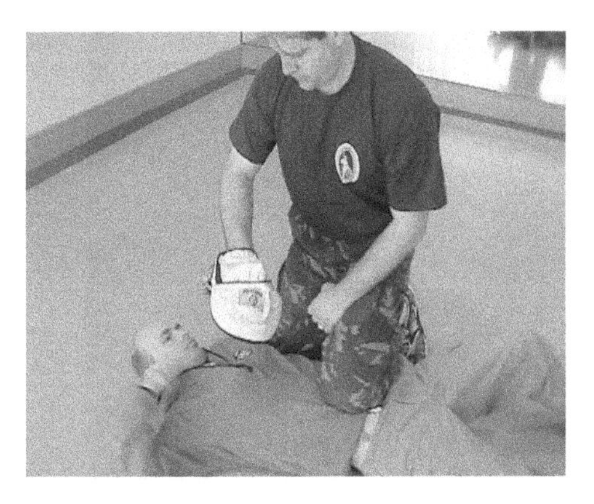

MOVING DRILLS

For these the pad holder is mobile, . taking steps forward and back. It is the hitters job to maintain range. The holder can also be moving the pads around between each strike. This allows the hitter to develop combinations and continuous striking methods. Remember to maintain appropriate position and angle on the pads.

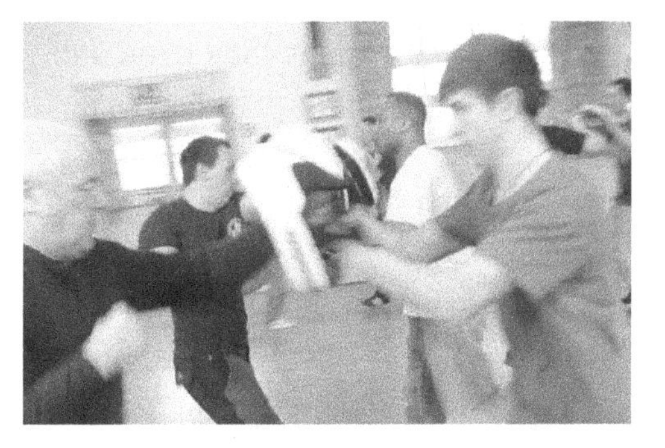

Work the same basic strikes but this time with added movement as described above.

Now let's try some reaction drills. The aim of these is to sharpen our reaction time while keeping our movements fluid and powerful.

Basic punch drill but the holder throws out occasional strikes with the pad. The hitter has to dodge them and return the hits.

Pad holder has hands at sides and suddenly brings the pad up into position for a second. The striker hits the pad as quick as possible.

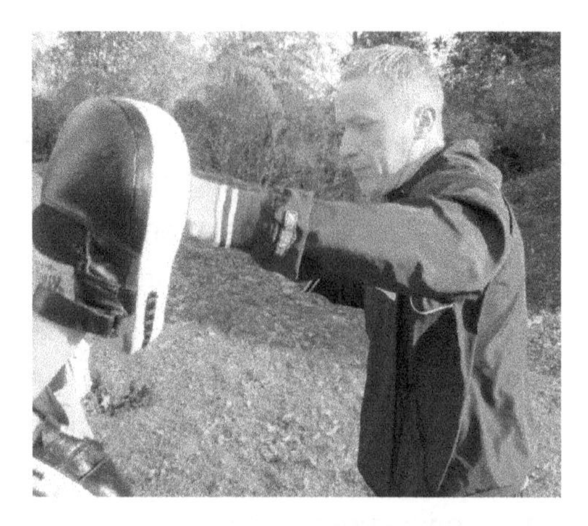

Hitter closes eyes. Pad holder positions the pad somewhere and says "go". The hitter opens their eyes and has to hit the pad as quickly as possible.

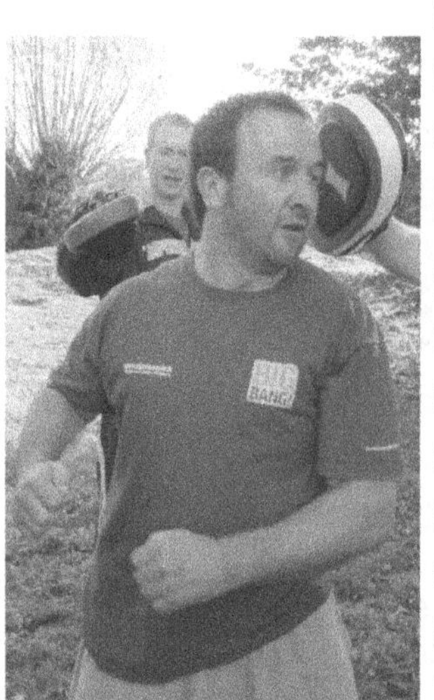

Pad holder hits the hitter with the pads then brings the pads into position. The hitter has hit back as quickly as possible.

Our next sequence of drills are to develop endurance and breathing. Experiment with different patterns while working, try burst breathing, pyramid breathing and so on while hitting. Also practice working with breath holds while hitting.

Start in basic punching position, with movement. After a certain interval the hitter has to transition through the levels - half squat, full squat, sitting and prone. Work a short time in each, then go back up to standing again. They have to keep hitting the pads throughout.

Ten seconds!
Establish a pattern of strikes. At the command "go!" the holder counts to ten while the hitter has to strike as fast as they can. Of course the count can be a slow ten....

2,4,6,8, 10
The holder shouts out one of the above numbers. That is the number of strikes the hitter has to do, as quickly as possible.

Elbows and knees
Pads are held at chest height for elbow strike. The hitter does three elbow hits

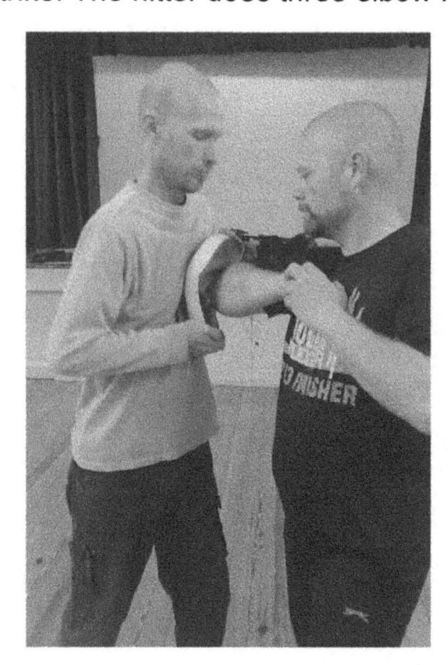

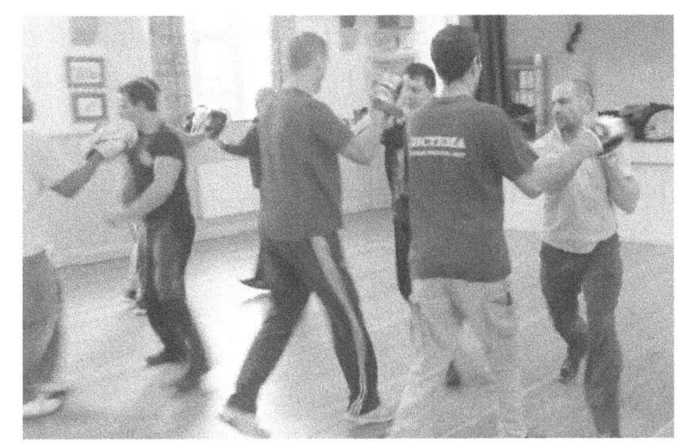

as fast as possible then pushes the pad holder away. The holder immediately transitions the pads to knee strike position. The hitter grabs the holder and does fast three knee strikes then pushes the holder back. Return to elbow position and repeat for a set time. The aim for the striker is to hit as hard and as fast as you can each time.

Chase and retreat
The pad holder either runs back at speed or pushes forward at speed. The hitter has to maintain distance while moving and striking.

GROUP DRILLS

These involve three or more people and are useful for learning to work against multiple attackers. We can also use this method for some types of pressure work.

Work the basic striking drills as before but with two or more pad holders and one striker. You can start with fixed, then go on to the pad holders moving. The hitter should be as fluid as possible with their striking. You can work in any of the restrictions from before and also adapt most of the pair exercises too.

As well as being hit we can also use the pads to hit! This is more of a

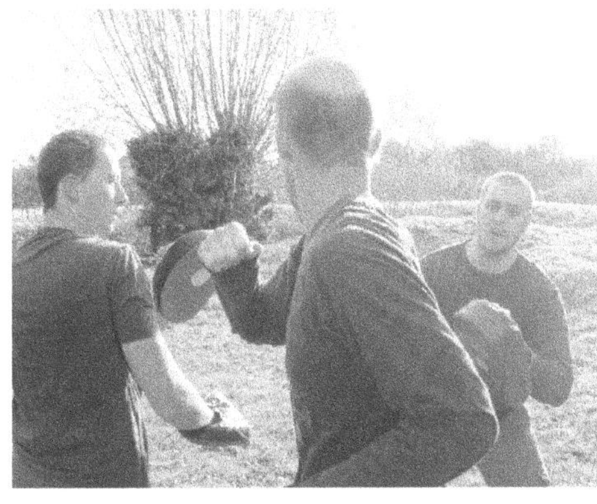

conditioning / fear control drill. One person stands in the middle of a circle of pad holders and must stain in place. The pad holders hit and slap the person for a set period of time.

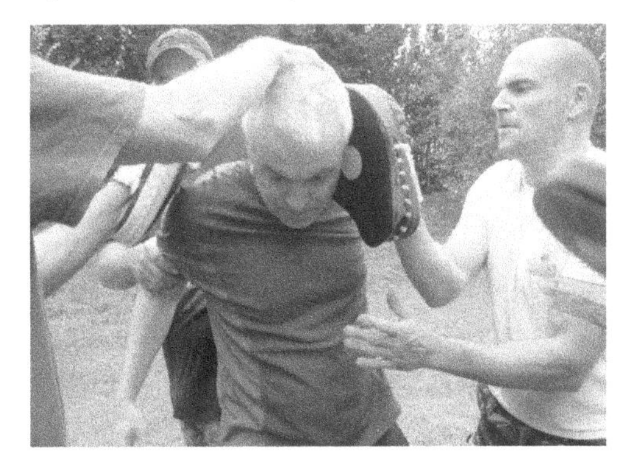

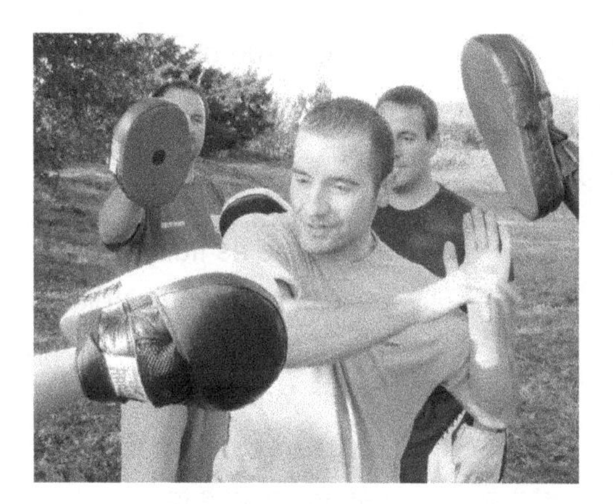

Intensity should be gauged according to the level of the person in the centre. Their goal is to use breathing and posture to maintain a steady psychological state. They are not allowed to move out of the circle or to retaliate in any way.

For a variation on the above, work the same drill but after a signal, the person in the centre begins hitting the pads as fast as they can. While doing so they should still maintain the same psychological state and general awareness.

KICK SHIELDS

We don't have to use just focus pads to hit, there are a range of different types of kick shields too.

If you want to work roundhouse-type kicks or knee strikes, PA positions the shield tight against their leg and PB performs the kick. PA can brace a little or, if the kick is very strong, relax the leg on impact to help absorb the strike. This same hip movement can be used for a

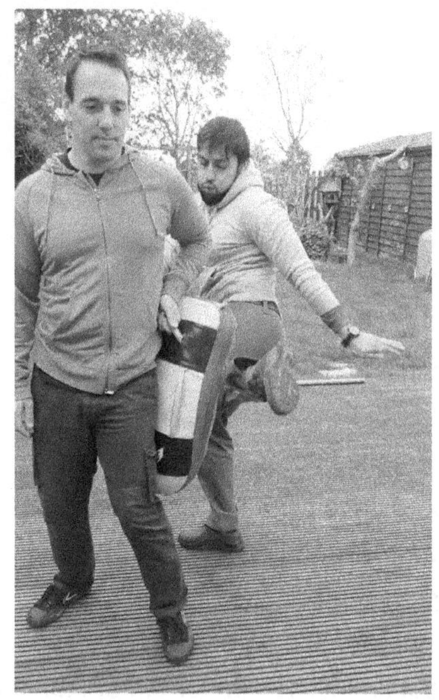

knee strike. In this case the kick shield can be held against the leg, or a little higher up to work different targets.

So to work any type of kick, simply place the shield at the appropriate position and angle. If you have a few shields, you can work in a more dynamic way. Have the group move the shields into different position, forcing the kicker to move, target and kick rather than work a static technique.

Kick shields can also be used in pressure testing. Have the group with shields pen PA in a corner and try and keep them there. PA has to escape, using any kind of strike, push or kick against the shields. You can work a similar idea but have PA pinned to the floor rather than in a corner

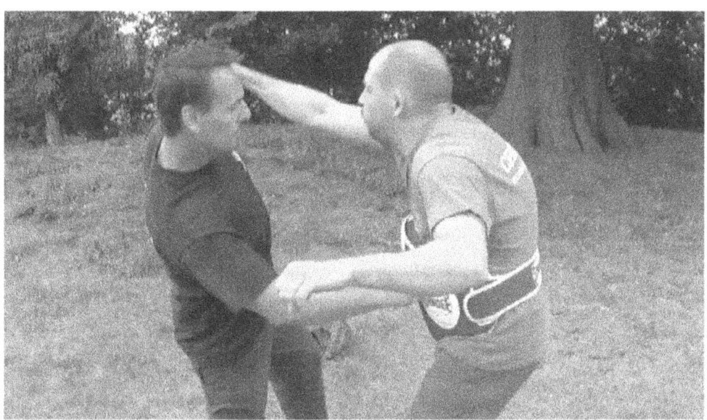

BODY ARMOUR

This is not something we use often and it usually relates more to sparring type drills or scenario work than exercise. However I will mention it here as it fits into the general field of "pads". Let's start with gloves.

Occasionally we will use light bag gloves for free style sparring work. This is to help protect the hands a little and allow everyone to work more freely. We never use boxing gloves as, I feel, they change the distance, shape of the fist and can be used as a shield when punching. All good things if you are training for the ring, but not so much for outside.

In fact I can think of only one drill where we use boxing gloves. PA is in the centre of the group wearing boxing gloves and a blindfold. The rest of the group push/slap PA around, PA has to relax. At the signal, PA begins swinging and must try to fight their way out of the group. Now PA is blindfolded so can be hitting anything, hence the use of large gloves for the sake of all concerned! This is more a psychological drill than a technical one.

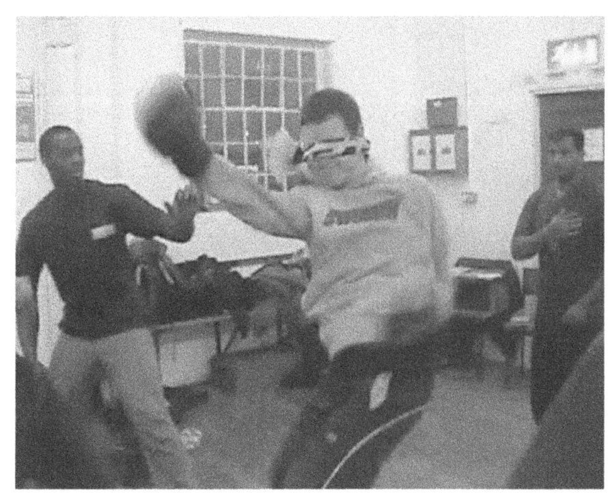

Other types of body armour include head gear and padding for the torso. Again, we occasionally use each from more freestyle work or if people want to really try out full power punches. We don' particularly use them while developing punches as, again, they change the dynamic. We do, though, advise the use of protective gear in certain types of weapons drill, especially eye protection.

Like everything, it is up to you to experiment and find out what works best with your group.

CHAPTER SEVEN
FALLS AND FLOOR

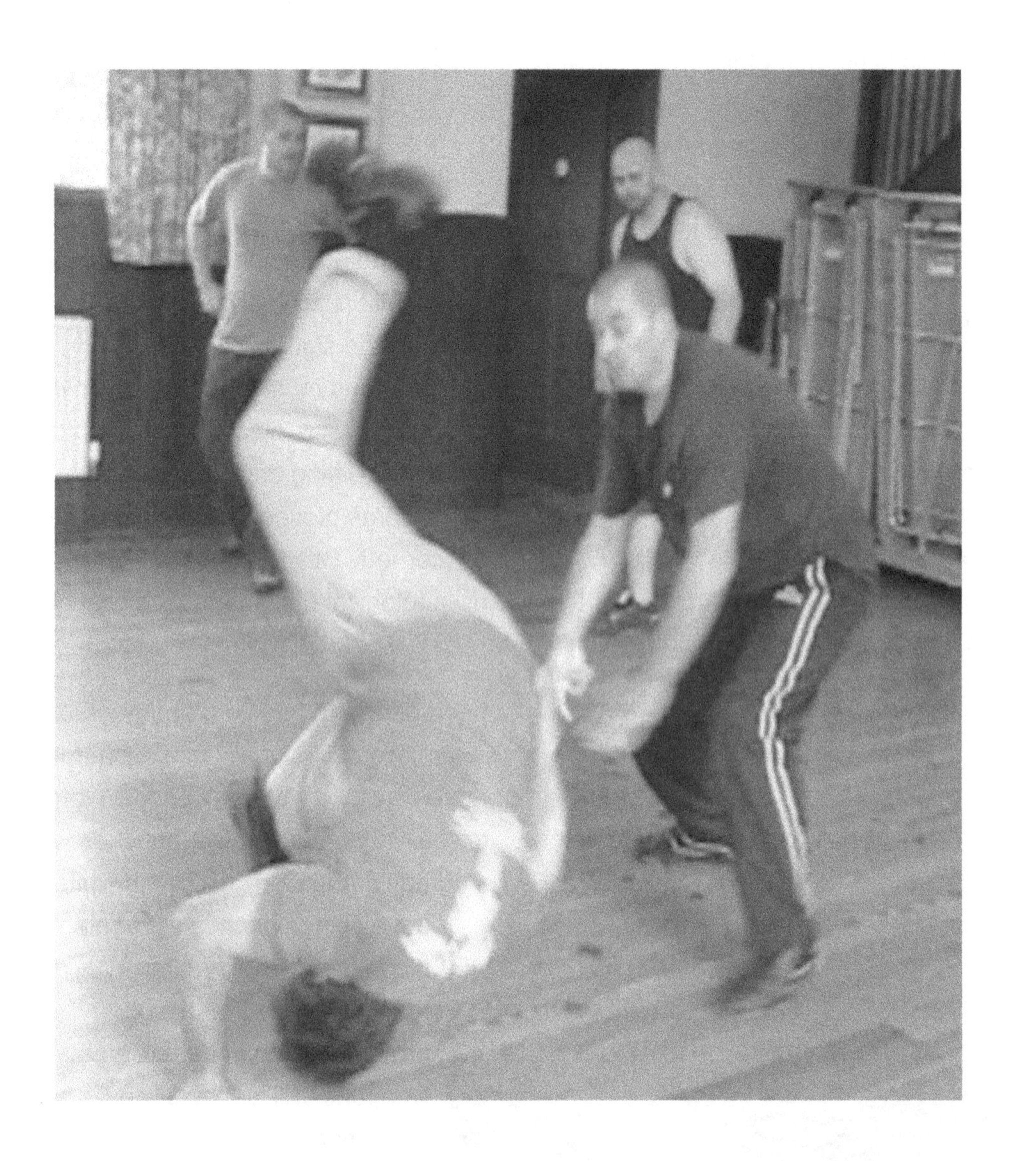

FALLS AND FLOOR

Falls and groundwork are one area where it is good to get a solid base in solo training before working with partners. Having said that there are many ways that a partner can help develop our basic skills, as well as working on more challenging exercises.

Using a partner to "assist" with falling takes away the control we have when working solo and so forces us to address the fear and tension that often comes with this work. As always, we advise beginning slowly and carefully, increasing intensity as skill levels progress. It is fine to use mates where necessary. It goes without saying that the key to falling safely is softness and breathing!

We will start with takedowns – I define this as collapsing a person's structure from in close in order to take them to the floor. From a static position, PA places hands on PB and affects a takedown. This should be soft at first and also give a clear direction of falling – ie do not twist or turn the faller just yet. PB's job is to go smoothly to the floor. Once there,

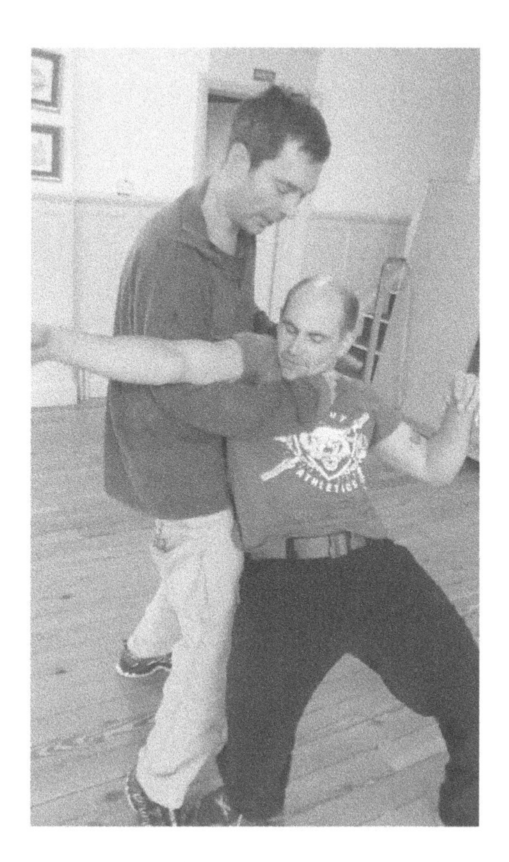

it is a good habit to develop moving away from the other person.

To make the exercise more challenging, PA can apply more speed to the takedown and also put some "twists" into their movement. This means PB's body will be forced to deal with more difficult trajectories.

Following this, we add in movement. Now PA and PB walk towards each other and, when in range PA carries out the takedown. Work through the same procedure as before. After a while, change the

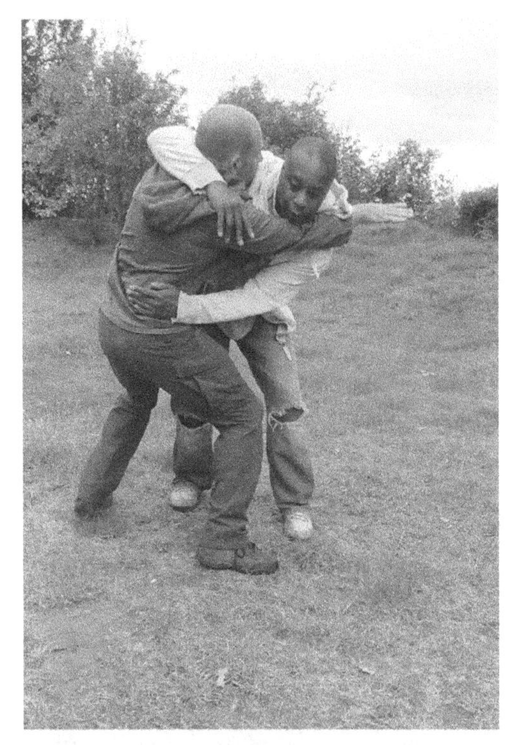

angles of approach. Once again, a blindfold adds an extra level of challenge.

Once everyone is fluid in being taken to the floor, we can begin to work on reversing takedowns. Start with the standing static exercise. This time, as PB is taken down they work to grab or hold PA in some way and take the person down with them. This should be done in such a way that leaves PB in an advantageous position. From this basic idea you can then work in the movement as above.

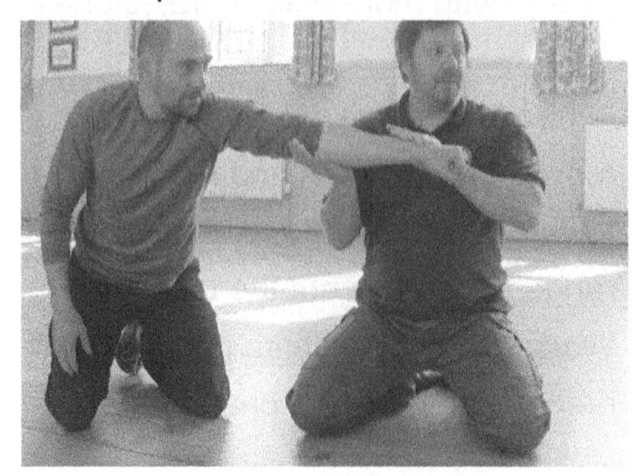

We can use the same approach to develop throws. Both partners kneel. PA takes PB's wrist and, using the leverage of the arm, "throws" them. As there is not so far to fall this allows PB to work on rolling out of a throw without fear.

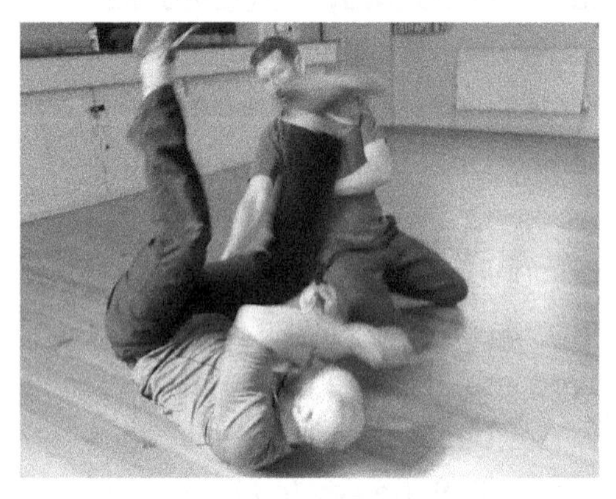

Once both partners have tried this, we can work on counter-throws. From the same position, as PB is thrown they work to take PA with them.

We now go to the standing static exercise. PB offers an arm or allows PA to clinch or hold the body. From here PA carries out any type of throw. PB goes with the movement and works to fall safely. At first the throw should be straightforward and

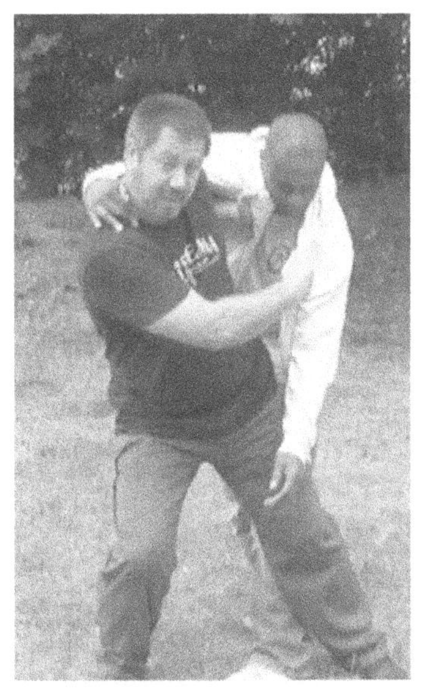

give a clear direction for the throwee. As skills increase, throws can be made more challeng ing.

The final level is again to add in the counter-movement. Both partners should be prepared for this, as it can be challenging work. Accept the throw and then work to throw your partner as you are moving in the air.

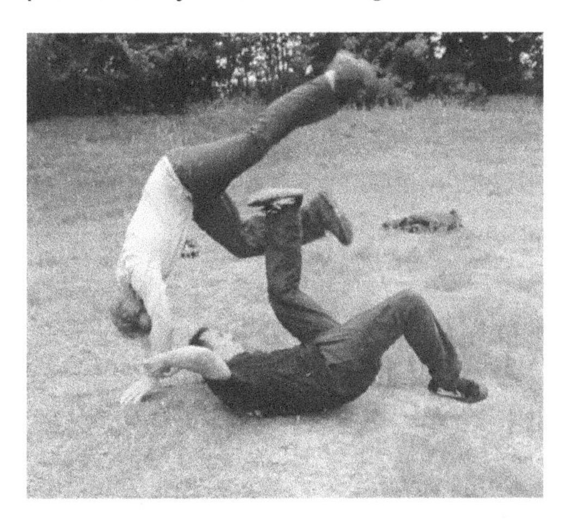

Let's also look at other partner work to help develop falls and rolling. This can be to deal with impact or to make an evasive maneuver. It helps to develop freedom and confidence and the body and teaches us a lot about impact management.

We start from standing position. PA pushes PB forward or back. PB takes a couple of steps and then falls and rolls to disperse the energy of the push. Pushes should be light at first, becoming heavier. For an added challenge PA can close eyes or wear a blindfold (be sure the area is free of obstacles).

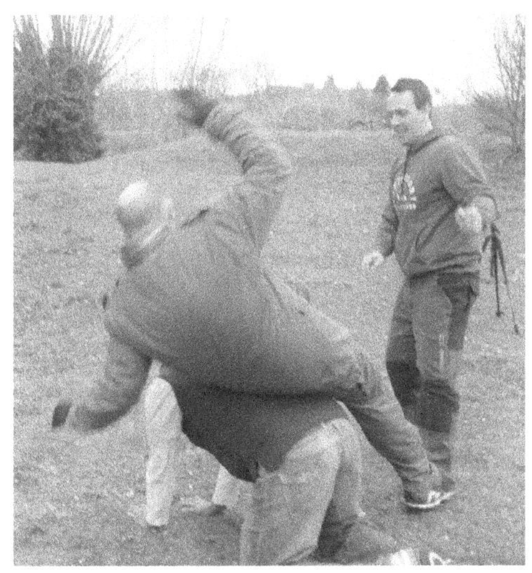

The next progression is to add in an obstacle. We suggest using another person at first, so welcome back PC! Here's the initial set up. PC kneels on all fours. PB stands close to PC and PA pushes PB, not too hard to start. PB has to fall softly over PC.

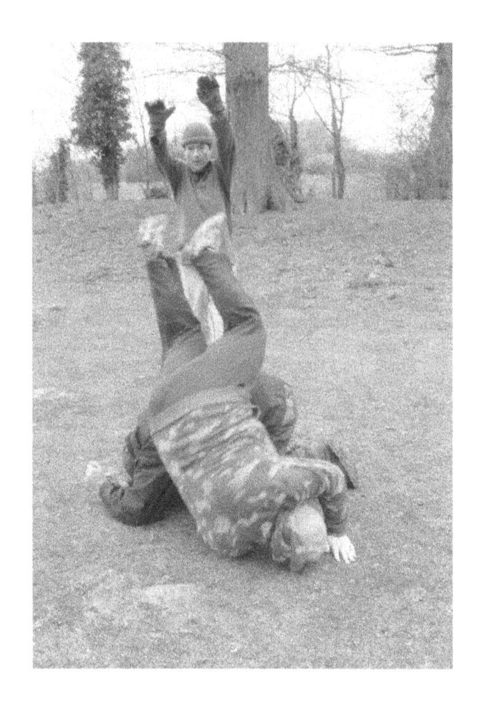

Once you have the basic idea, you can increase the distance and the strength of the push. Eventually, PB should be diving over PC. Following this you can use other objects, a chair, a bench or so on, as the obstacle. Our most challenging was a moving car but that is an exercise only to be tried under supervision!

Now we are on the ground, we have to learn how to move there! The simplest exercise is to work in pairs. PA is on the ground and PB walks towards them, giving a single line of direction (ie don't track PA). All PA has to do is avoid contact.

Begin with clear, large movements. PA can either move to increase distance from PB, or work to stay on the spot, using minimal movement to avoid contact.

As the drill progresses PA can apply more speed, quicker changes of direction and so on. To add in an extra level, PB can work to take down PA at some point.

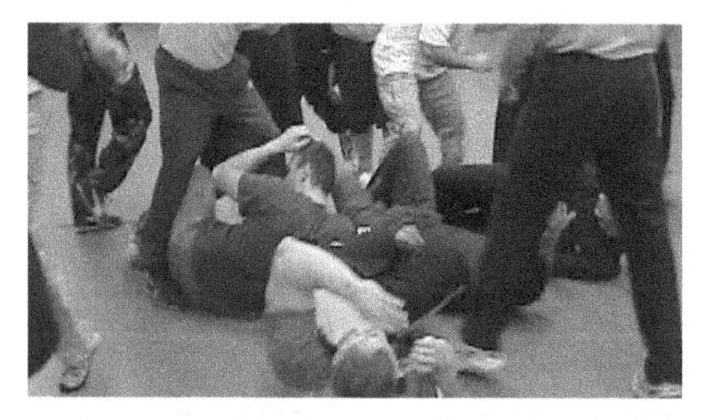

If you want to work a larger group, you can use the Zombie drill from earlier. The person on the floor is now the target of the "walkers". In fact, with a large group you can have two or more people on the floor avoiding the walkers. At a signal they can work to take a walker down, get up and switch roles.

If you want to work in more pressure, go back to the partner drill and instead of PB walking, they try and step on or kick PA. Once again, we start with clear, slow movements and progress from there. PA can attempt to avoid contact or carry out a takedown.

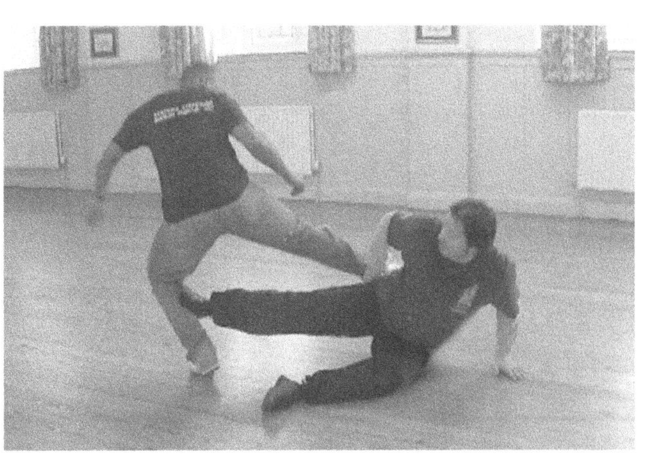

When both partner's are confident, try this drill. The set up is as above, PA on the floor, PB kicking or stamping. PA carries out the takedown and must get up as quickly as they can. Immediately, they then try and kick and stamp on PB, who now does the takedown and gets up quickly. Repeat for as often as you like, try and maintain smoothness and speed.

Returning to our large group, a good fear inoculation drill is to have one or more people on the floor while the rest of the group "fights" above them. This is one way to replicate being on the floor in a crowd, where there is no direct focus on you but nonetheless there is real risk present. At a signal, those on the floor can either get up quickly or takedown a crowd member in order to switch positions.

For another fear control drill, have PA lay on their back and PB kneel over them. PB then has to fall directly onto PA who must manage the impact.

Another version of this drill is to learn to cope with an even heavier weight!. This time PA lays on the floor, front and back. Three, four or five people then take it in turns to slowly lay on PA, building up a "stack"of people. PA should work breathing and position to hold their place for a while, then they can move out from under the group as smoothly

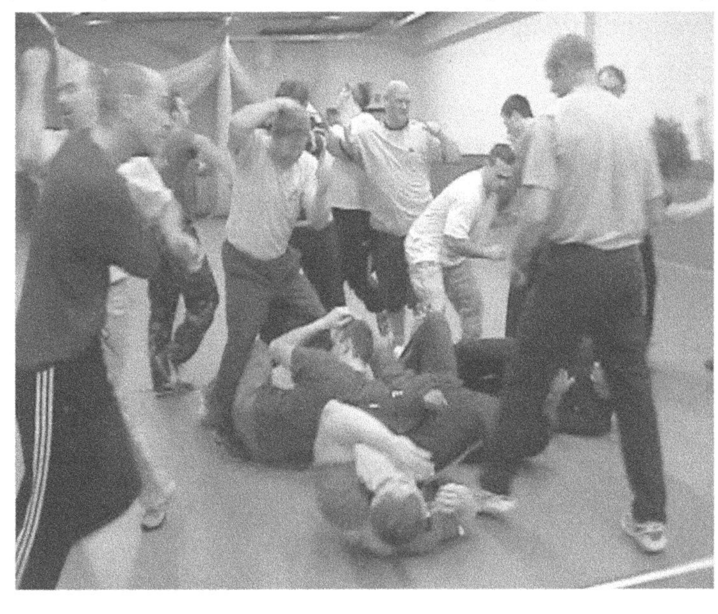

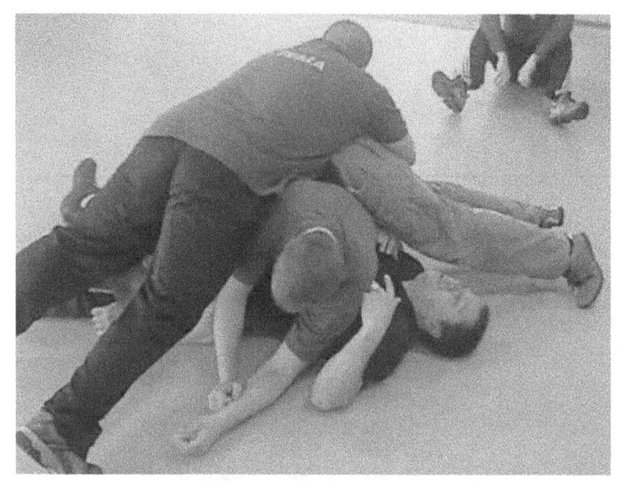

as possible. We strongly advise having one person monitoring this drill, at any sign of difficulties from PA the other people should immediately get up.

There are several ways we can work with others to improve our ground movement. One easy drill is to have PA in raised push up position. PB has to move in, under, over and through PA as smoothly as possible.

Another method is to go through

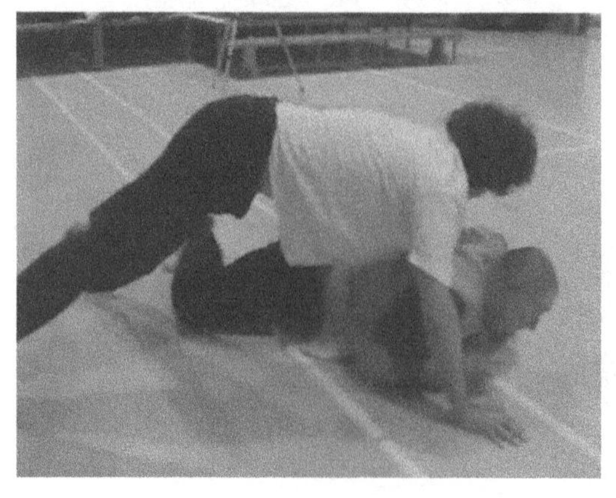

the solo movement exercises while carrying another person. For example, PA lays face down and can only use their arms in order to move. PB lays across their back as a dead weight. Repeat in different positions and using different parts of the body to move.

With a larger group, keep everyone in the centre of the training

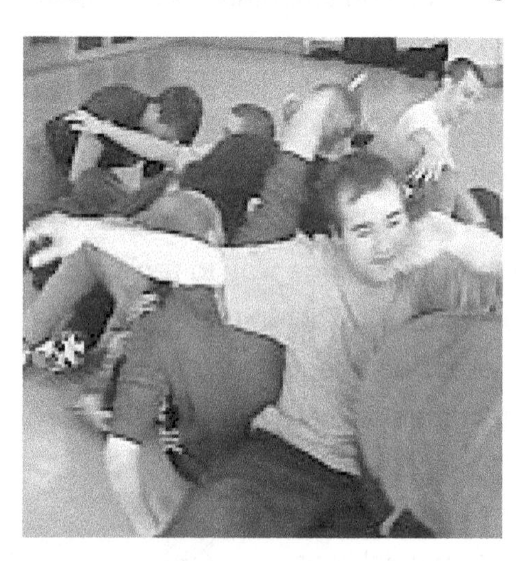

space and have them move around. They can either work to avoid contact as much as possible or to move directly on and over the other people.

Returning to pairs, PA now carries out forward or backward rolls, while PB restricts their movement. This done by at first having PB stand

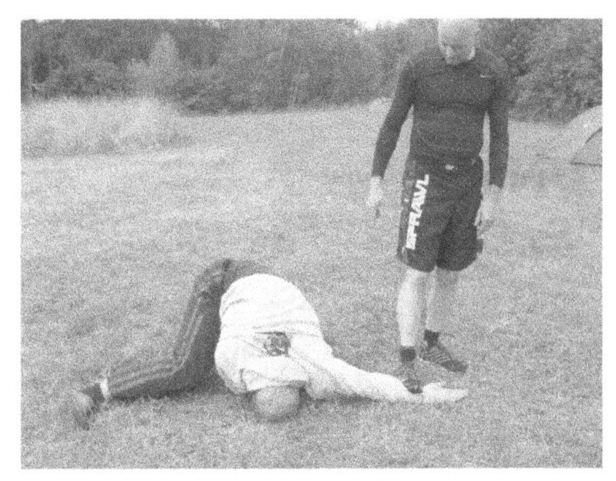

on PA's wrist, pinning it to the floor. Following this, PB steps on the elbow and finally the shoulder. Repeat on the other side, then switch roles. You can try this same idea while pinning other parts of the body.

Another idea is for partners to roll in unison. You can link arms or hold hands and carry out forward and backward rolls. You can start from kneeling or work from standing.

You can add in more people, work in threes, fours and so on. With a larger group, have everyone stand in a circle and link arms or place arms over shoulders. At a signal, the whole group goes to the floor onto their backs. Repeat, with everyone going onto their fronts (with care!).

We will conclude this section with one last falling drill. This one is challenging and should only be practiced by experienced students. I also advise using mats to begin with. This drill originates with a military method to simulate jumping from a moving vehicle.

Four people hold PA by the wrists and ankles. At the signal they lift PA off the ground and begin to swing PA back and forward on a count. On the count of three, PA is released at the top of the arc to sail through the air and land gracefully! You can start by keeping PA a little lower. It is hard to go slow as the exercise relies on momentum, but take some care at first. With experience and skill you will be surprised at how far and high you can launch someone and they can manage the landing!

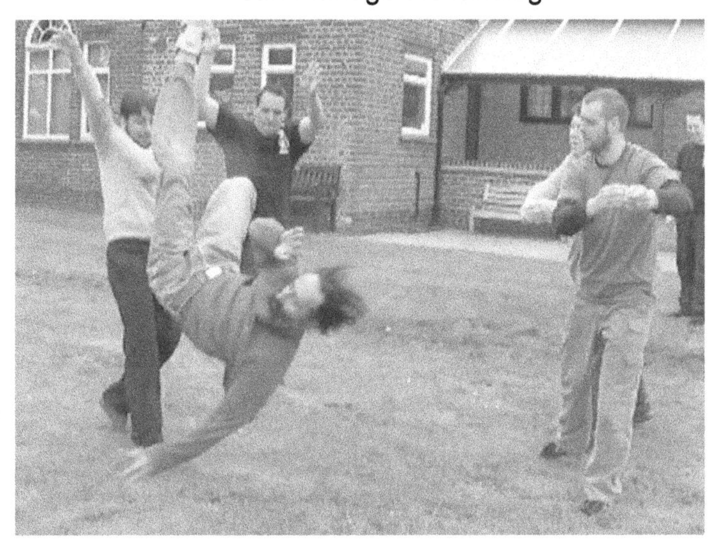

CHAPTER EIGHT
WEAPONS

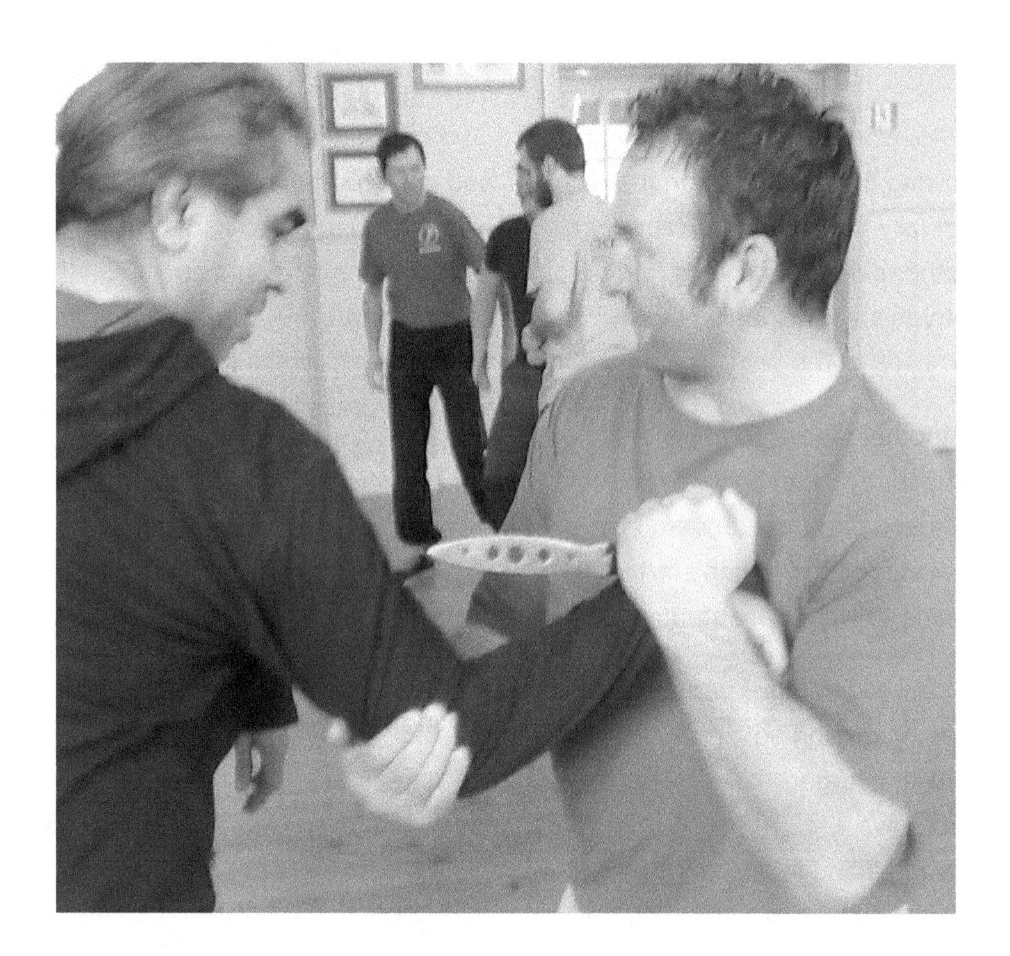

WEAPONS

As we mentioned in the Solo Training book, learning the proper use of weapons is something that should be done under the supervision of qualified instructors.

However, as we also mentioned, there are many simple ways to utilise weapons purely as tools to help develop various skills and attributes. Some are universal, others are specific to a certain weapon. Again, we are working here on the attribute development role, be it movement, awareness or sensitivity, rather than any tactical considerations. Let's start with some universal drills.

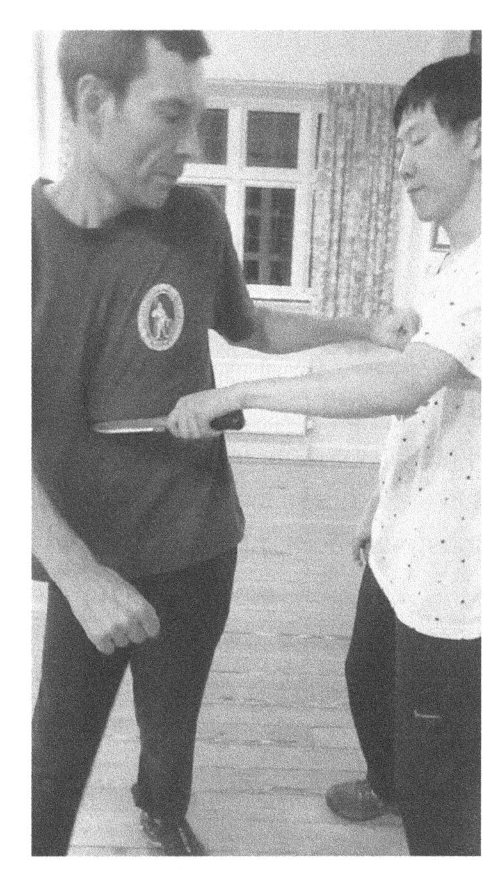

PA pushes PB with the weapon. It can be a stick, knife gun, the procedure is the same. PB accepts the push and moves away from it, either as a whole body movement or just the area pushed. There are numerous variations - have two or more people pushing, both partners push each other simultaneously, the pushee can be blindfolded and you can adjust positions, go to the floor, sit down and so on.

You can develop these exercises into disarming drills and from there develop into flow drills. Check our book The Ten Points of Sparring for more ideas.

Along similar lines, PA works pre-contact and attempts to avoid contact with the weapon. All the same variables can be added in.

Carry and draw drills can be done with most weapons, or at least those small enough to be concealed about the person. We start in pairs.

PA faces away from PB who hides the weapon on their person. At a signal, PA turns and as quickly as possible finds and removes the

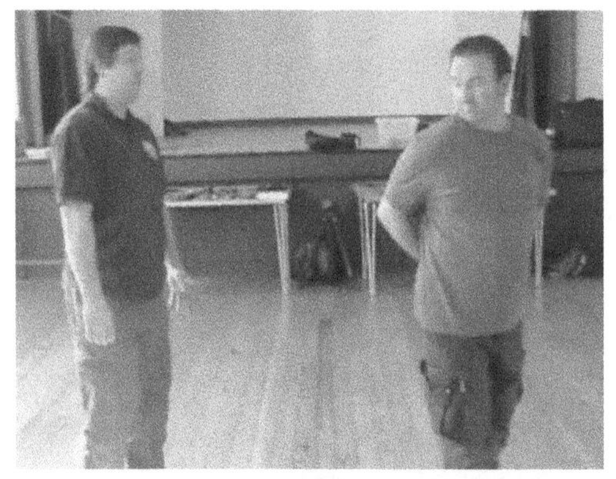

weapon. To progress this drill, as PA turns, PB draws the weapon. PA must work quickly to jam the draw.

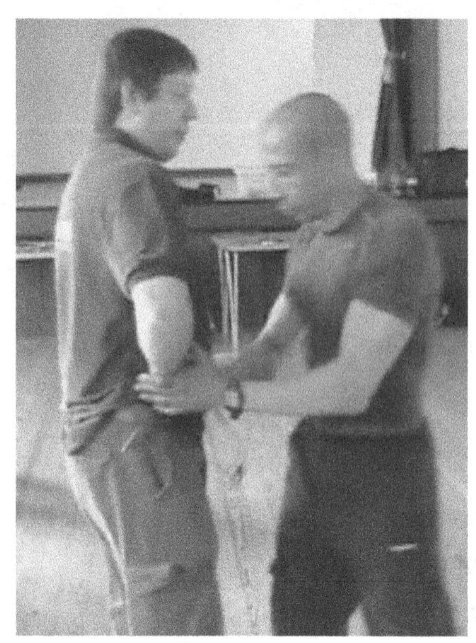

These drills can be translated to group work too. You can have the group stand in a line, one person secretly conceal the weapon while PA looks away. As before, PA turns and must spot the weapon as quickly as possible. You can progress along same lines as the pair drill. You can also add in movement. Have more than one person in the group conceal. The group then all move around and everyone tries to spot who is carrying the weapons.

The next stage is the draw. The weapon holder/s can draw at any time, at which the rest of the group must quickly go to the floor, move under cover and/or move in to disarm the wielder

Now let's look at some more specific exercises. The first is designed to improve reaction time and ground movement. PA lays faces up. PB holds a knife over them at shoulder height. Now of course this should be a training knife, we suggest a rubber one to start!

PB counts out loud 1, 2, 3 and drops the knife on three. PA has to

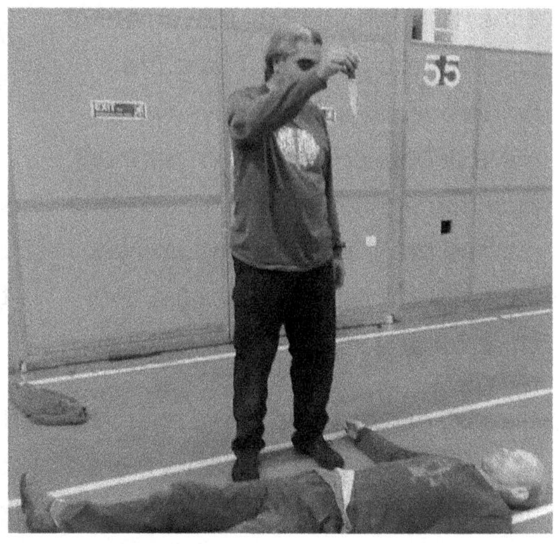

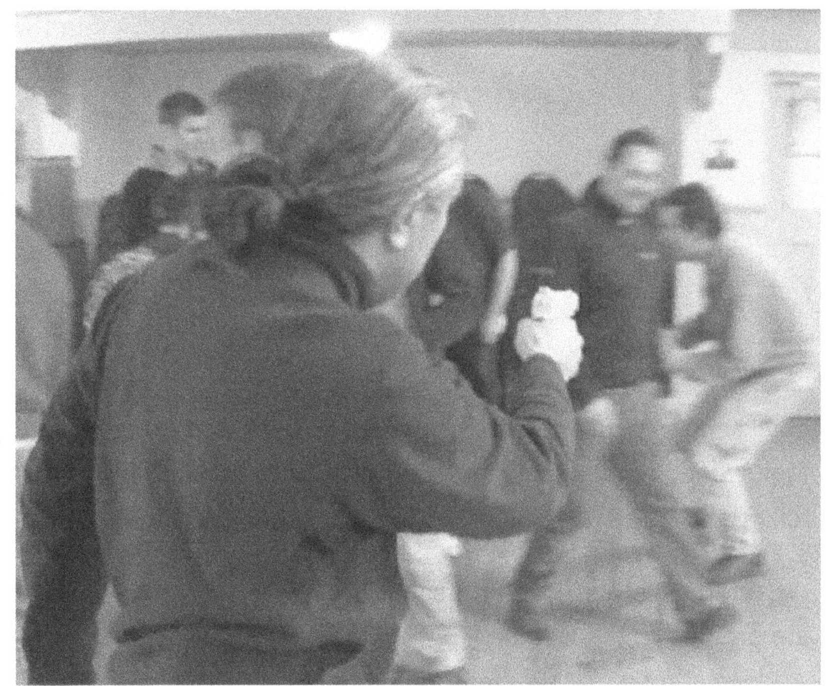

avoid it as it falls. Run through a few times, then move on to the next stage. Now PB drops on a count of one. For the final stage PB makes no count at all, just drops the knife.

You can further increase the challenge by holding the knife lower to start. If you feel uncomfortable using a knife, you can do the same exercise with a tennis ball or similar.

The gun can be used to good effect for movement and awareness drills. As there is no firing involved, you can use a rubber gun or anything you feel comfortable with. Let's start with simple pointing.

PA has the gun and has to continually keep it pointed at PB. Both are moving around and can change level, hide behind obstacles and so on. It is quite interesting to do this in pairs but involving a large group. This means you have to track your "target" in amongst a crowd.

As a variation start with the same set up but give everyone a gun. Have the gun holders switch targets every now and then. All the people in the group now have to be aware if they are a target as well as watching their own target.

Going back the draw drills, we can work in some more variations. Have everyone in the group moving around with a holstered gun. One other person, unarmed, also moves around and at some point claps their hands. The rest of the group must

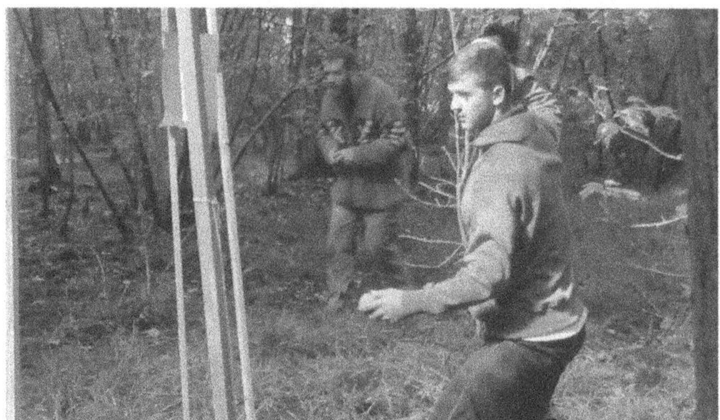

quickly go to the floor while drawing their weapon and aiming it at the "clapper".

Alternatively we can arm some of the group with tennis balls. Either working in rows, facing the throwers, or in a random group, the gun holders must evade a thrown tennis ball whilst drawing the gun and aiming it at the thrower.

Of course once you get into airsoft training there are a whole range of firearm drills you can work with, but that is beyond the scope of this book. So let us now move on to working with the chain.

There are a few simple exercises we can work in pairs with a chain. The chain should be reasonably heavy and about three or four feet long. The chain is a great tool for developing softness in the body as any tension in the wrong place will prove painful!

Start with partners facing each other. PA rests the chain across their forearms, PB stands in a similar position. PA tosses the chain to PB who catches it with a yielding movement on their forearms. Work back and forth, static at first, then you can begin moving around and, changing level.

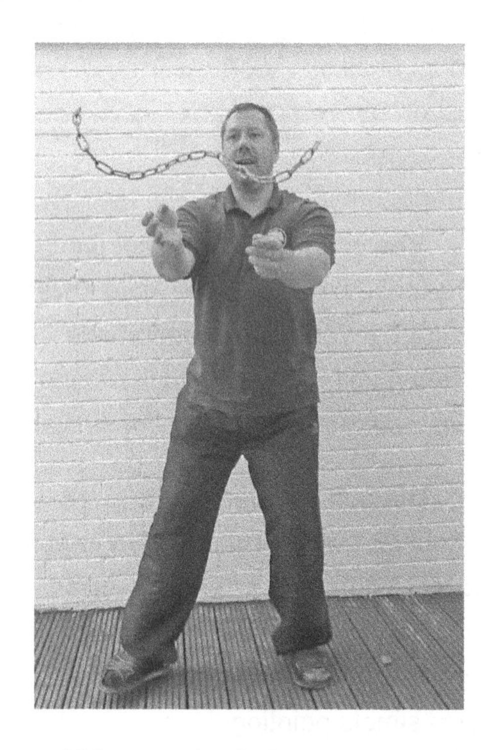

This exercise helps us get used the impact of the chain. For the next stage, PA stands with arms outstretched. PB holds the chain at one end and swings it either under or over PA's arm. On impact PA rotates

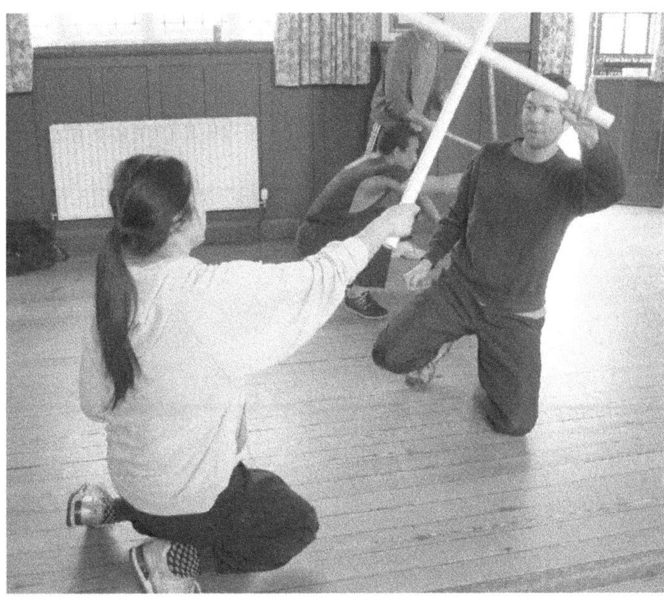

the arm in order to absorb the impact of the chain. Once you have the feel for the arms, work with the chain striking the body. It is important with these drills that the chain is swung with a reasonable amount of force. Too weak and there is little benefit from the exercise. Of course, it should not be too hard at first, but with time you can learn how to deal with a strong swing.

Another variation of the arm rotation drill is for PA to "flick" the chain back on impact. PB needs to work to avoid the return! You can also try the same method using the legs.

We also covered sword work in our previous book and, of course there are many sparring partner drills that can be done. These range from repeating a few set movements to free play and sparring. In terms of purely attribute development, sensitivity work is one of the most useful.

PA and PB face each other and make light contact with the swords, or, of course you can use metal blades, training / wooden swords or plastic pipes.

PA now slowly moves and PB has to try and maintain blade contact. Add in level changes, increase speed, etc as required. To progress, have one partner attempting to touch the other with the blade. The sensitivity now becomes more active. Switch roles, then finally both can attack and defend, but always maintaining contact.

With a little thought it is easy to convert the same drill to other weapons - the stick, knife shovel, etc. Of course you don't have to match weapons - give one partner a knife, the other a stick! Again, be creative!

CHAPTER NINE
ATTRIBUTES

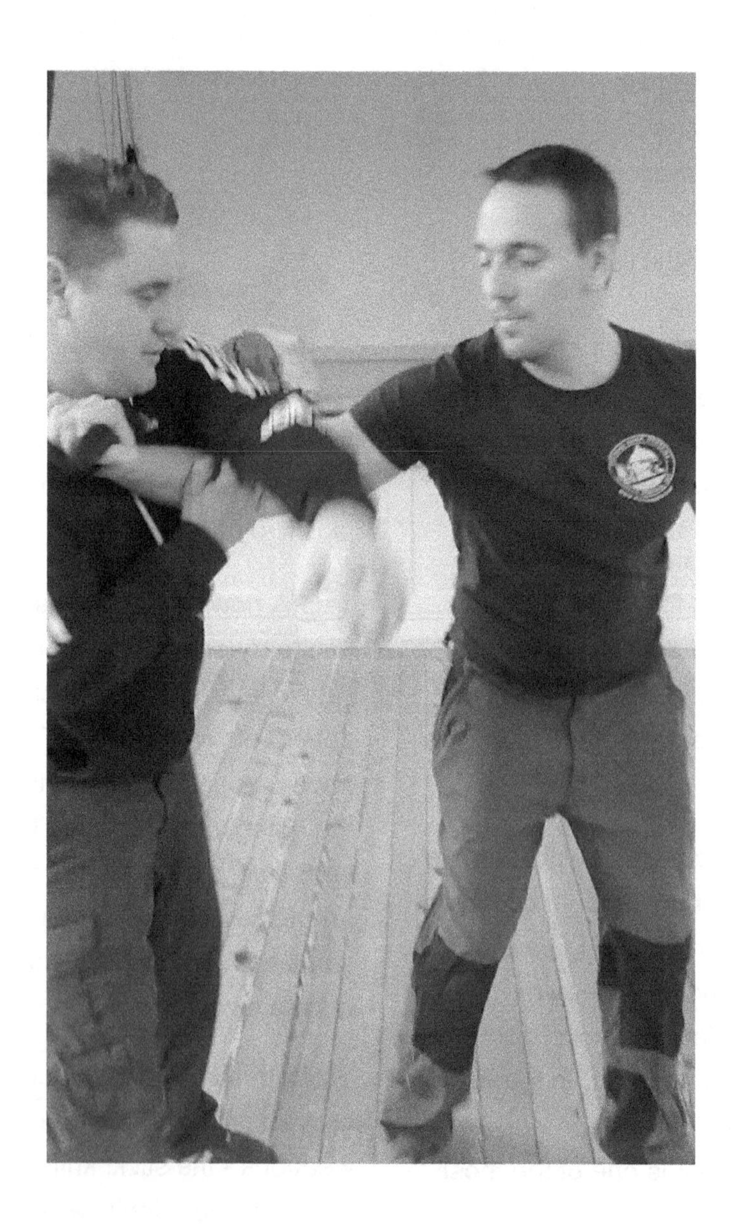

ATTRIBUTES

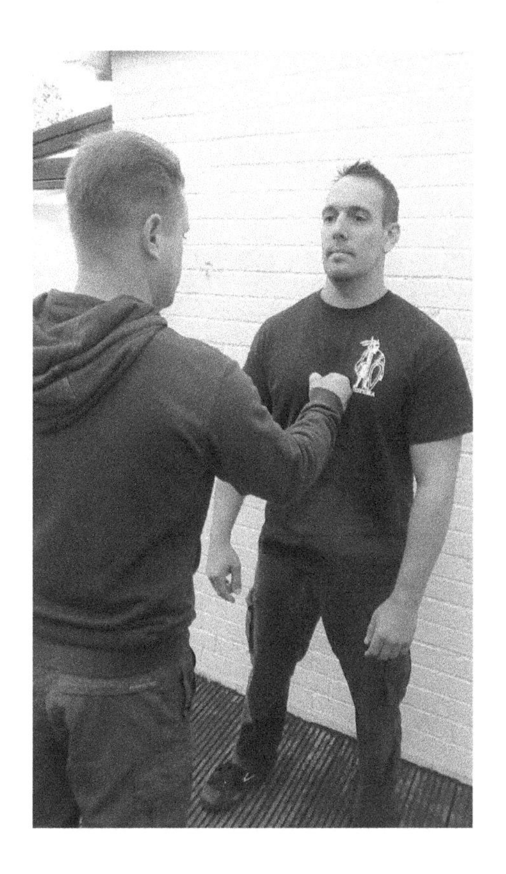

The following exercises are put under the general heading of Attributes. They are not directly strength building exercises as such but nor are they combat drills. What they are designed to do is to develop a wide range of skills and attributes, such as sensitivity, balance, awareness, fear control and so on. These can then be incorporated into you combat practice in order to increase your efficiency. Of course they can also be practiced purely for enjoyment and developing different types of movement, the function is up to you.

Most of these drills have numerous layers that are added in as people progress and can also be combined together in some cases. As always, the possibilities are almost endless. Systema is an open ended training method, not a collection of techniques or movements. We will start with basic drills to develop body softness and sensitivity.

PA pushes PB with a closed fist. It should be a reasonably strong push. The aim for PB is to allow the contact and then go with the movement - you allow your partner to push you. Your body can respond in two ways. You can move the whole body in the direction of the push, so if pushed back you take a step or two back to absorb the force. Or you can move just the point of contact. So say your are pushed on the left shoulder, you roll just the shoulder to absorb the force. Try and exhale as you move away.

This is one of the fundamental Systema drills and appears in almost every class we teach. There are numerous variations from this starting point, here's are few ideas.

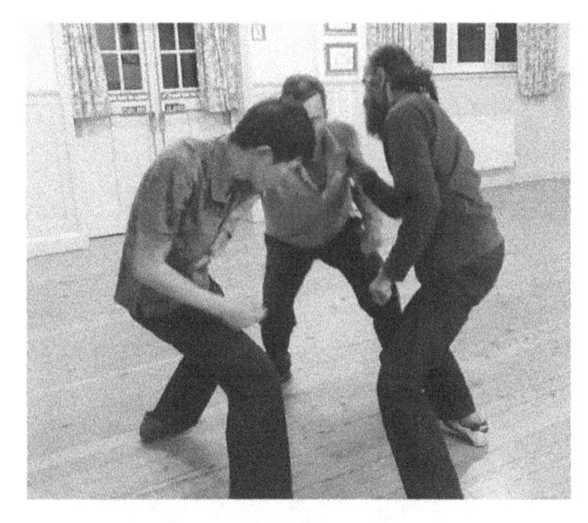

Partners push each other simultaneously. Try and use the movement from your partner's push in order to make your own push.

Work in groups of three or more. You can all push each other,or place one person in the middle and have

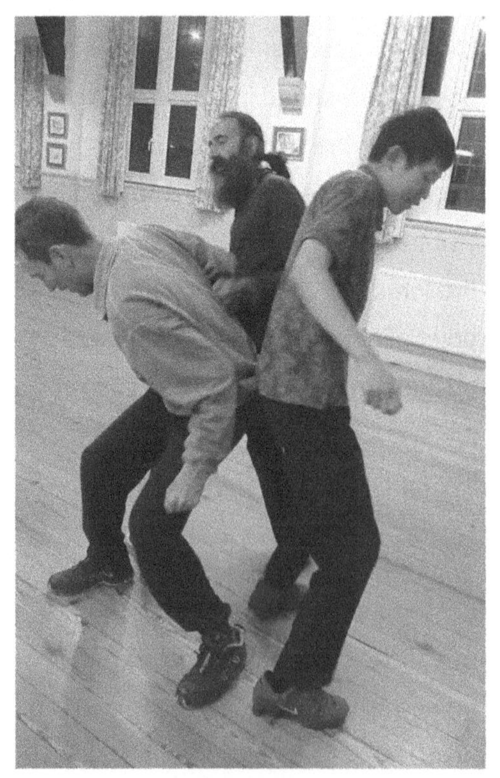

everyone push them.

The group gets into a circle, feet touching. Everyone pushes each other and tries to stay in the circle. Face inwards, then repeat with everyone facing outwards.

Work in different positions. Start standing, then transition into squat, seated and prone. Do not break the flow of movement as you change levels.

Work with the whole group. Everyone walks around the room and pushes whoever is closest. You can open up or restrict the space.

The same work can be done with strikes instead of pushes. Indeed, one function of the pushing is to prepare both partners for strike work.

Rather than a fist, push with the foot. This is obviously preparation for kicking work.

Now let's try the same, but working pre-contact. The basic method has become known as the Zombie Drill. Work in a group, one person is the target. The rest of the group try and walk into that person. They are not

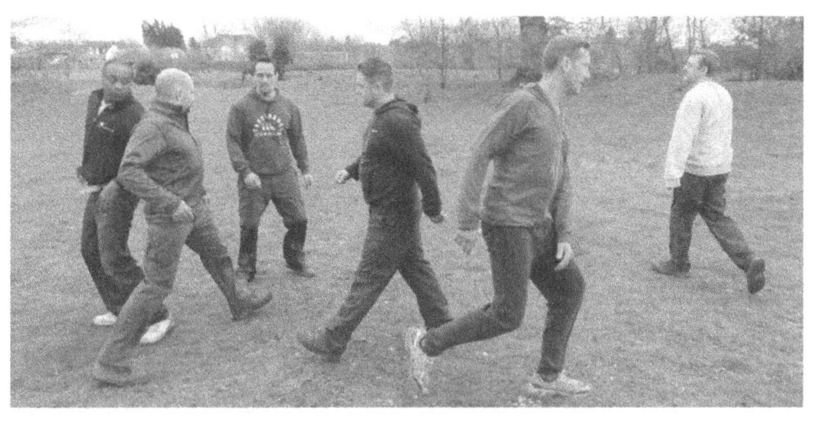

allowed to track, just walk in a straight line through the person. The target has to avoid contact with the "zombies". Keep your form and keep breathing, try to maintain all round awareness with peripheral vision. Speed can be varied as well as space available.

The next variation is the Dalek Drill. This is the same set up as before, but this time the walkers have a fist extended out in front of them.

GAUNTLET DRILLS

We have already looked at gauntlet drills with the stick, let's run through some ideas for empty hand gauntlet.

Position for the group is either a column (people stood one behind the other) or in rows (two lines face each other). The task for PA is to move from one end to the other. So each of the following will be described as C, column or R.row. The gaps between people can and should be varied. Shorter gaps can make for less space to move but they also shorten the line! Contact levels should also be varied, along with speed and intensity.
PA can move by walking, running, crawling, duck walk, etc

C. PA moves from end to end as smoothly as possible avoiding contact with the group. Repeat but have the group outstretch a fist or foot. Repeat again but have the group throw a punch or kick as PA approaches.

C. The aim is to take a strike but continue to move fluidly through. PA moves end to end, each person punches as they go past. Repeat with kicks. Repeat both with PA as the striker and the group as receivers. Repeat once more with both sides giving and taking strikes

R. Repeat both the above, strikes

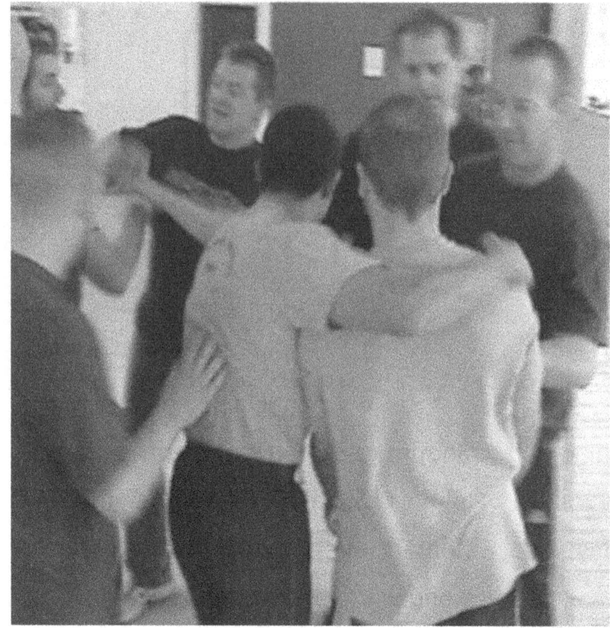

versions, with group in a row.
It is easy to repeat all these drills with weapons.

For a variation you can try this Close Protection drill. PA has now to guide PB through the gauntlet and try to prevent any of the group from touching PB. All the same variables can be applied.

As we have mentioned CP drills, let's look at some more. They are fun to do and teach us a lot about positioning, timing and psychology! People sometimes ask why we do CP drills when we are not (for the most part) bodyguards? My reply is that we are bodyguards every time we are out with our children, family, friends and so on. Be broad in your thinking, training is for your whole life, not just the time you are in the gym!

The basic drill is for PA and PB to stand close to each other. PA must attempt to remain in touching distance and move around PB smoothly. It should be possible to go from behind PB to in front of them in no more than two steps. The movement, or course, should be fluid and releaxed.

From here, PA is now static and moves PB around them. So you might

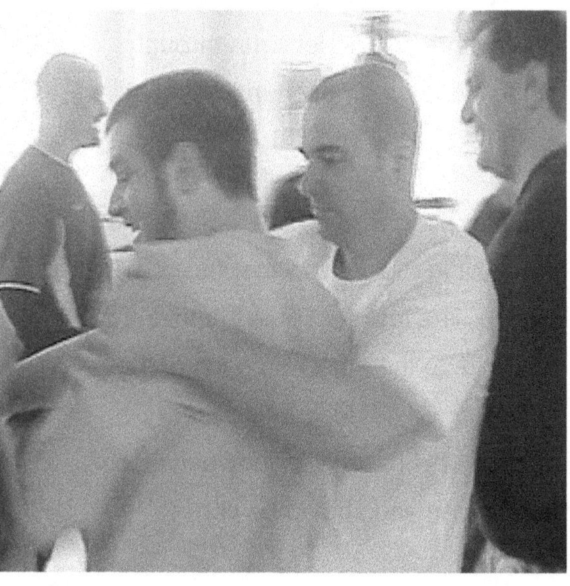

pull on the arm, push on a hip and so on. The movement should not be unpleasant for PB, after all this may be a paying client!

The next step is for PA to take PB smoothly and with as little impact as possible to the floor. Imagine you have to move the person out of the way of danger. You then also try the same work laterally, ie moving PB completely out of the immediate area.

Once all these are done, it is time to bring back PC, this time as the bad guy! We start wit the set up of PA behind PB. PC approaches from a distance away. PA has to move in front of PB and deal with the "threat". This can be done in a few ways. PA can softly re-direct PC with a deflecting touch. Then can try re-directing without contact, point, smile, present a barrier to the eyes or groin. They can do a takedown / restraint on PC. Or, of course, they can just hit them. Each is to reflect a different type of situation.

The next version is for PA to move PB out of the path of and way from PC. This can be a lateral movement or going to the floor. If you want to combine this with the earlier pistol

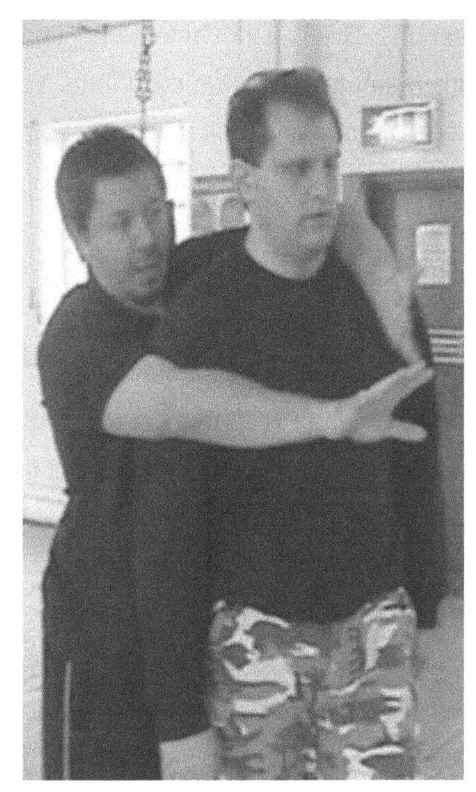

drills, have PA draw and aim as they move/shield PB.

These basic drill outlines can further be varied by adding in one or more extra "bodyguards". They have to work in synch so it is best that each is assigned specific roles. For example, one moves PB to safety while the other engages the threat. From here you can move into all types of scenario training and again we suggest looking at the Ten Points of Sparring book for pointers on how to do that.

Let's leave the CP world with one

last drill. This is a movement /reaction drill rather than a "protection" one. You need a group of people and a long length of rope or twine. PA and PB take and end of the rope each and stand at the end of the training area, one on each side of the room. The group stand randomly around the room. PA and PB stretch the rope out between them and run the length of the room. The group must either avoid contact with the rope and/or fall quickly to the floor. The rope can be held at different heights. You can also add in the "draw weapon" component or the "take down a friend" component - or both!

We touched on teamwork just now and in our earlier carrying drills, , so let's now look at some group drills designed to develop team awareness and communication skills.

PA stands close to PB and places a hand on them. PB moves around and PA must maintain contact. Speed, position, etc can all be varied.

PA stands behind PB with hands on their shoulders. PB closes their eyes and begins to walk around the room. PA must guide PB with touch only. The aim is to avoid contact with other pairs, walls, furniture, etc. Repeat but this time there is no contact, only verbal communication.

Once you have this basic idea established, you can work in larger groups. At first, simply have a line of people with hands on shoulders following the person at the front at a walk, jog or run.. The best way to keep movements in synch is through the breathing. Get the group to establish a square breathing count and move in

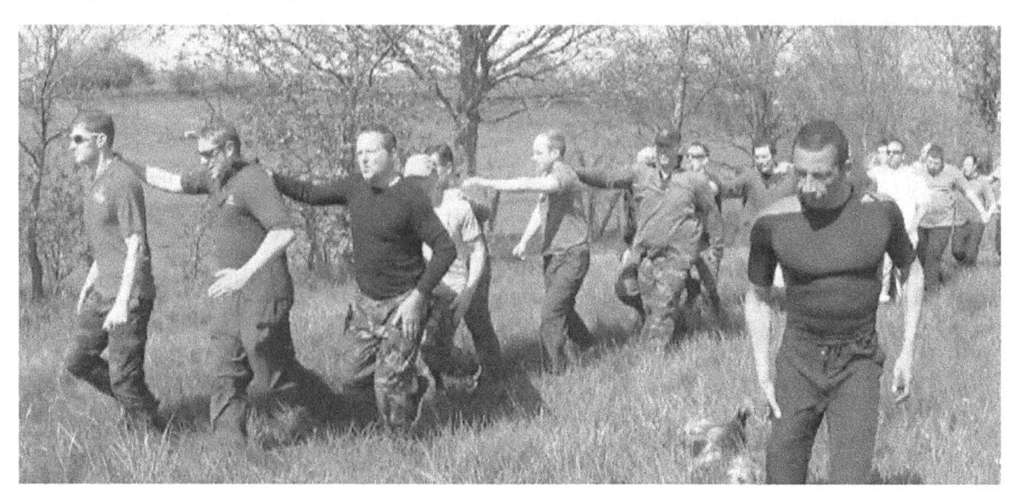

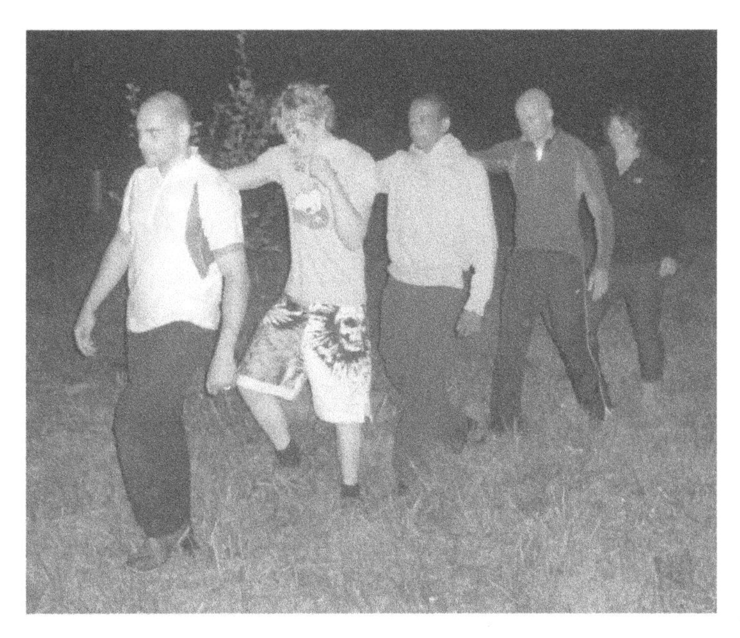

time with it. The can also slap the leg on every other step, for example.

From there, the group works "blind" and the person at the back steers. So now the communication must travel along the line. You can suggest ideas to the group or have them work out their own methods of communication.

You can have the group walk around the training room, with or without obstacles, This is also a great drill to do outside, with uneven ground, through trees and so on. We often run it during nighttime training as it develops trust in the group and ability to move in low light. Experiment with who has their eyes closed, different communication methods and so on. You can also easily add in obstacles or tasks and, of course, have two or more teams to race in order to increase pressure.

Eyes closed or blindfold work is a great method of developing sensitivity and intuition. Some of these exercises are physical and some are psychological. Systema is very much about developing our natural skills and intuition, something that tends to get buried in the fast moving world of technology. Even getting out into woods or fields for a walk can help but

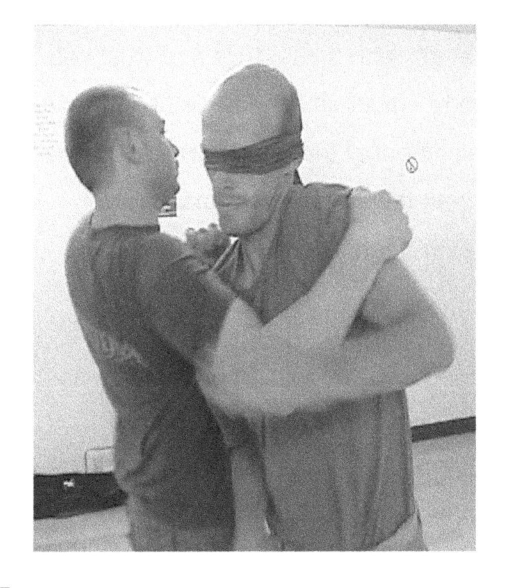

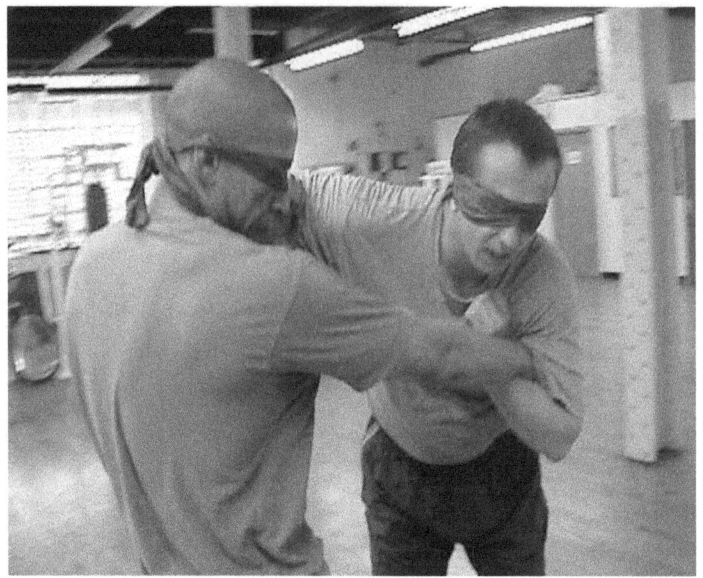

there are also some specific drills to reconnect us to our natural intuitive state.

We start with a simple physical drill, the pushing from earlier. Repeat any of the push, takedown or throwing drills with the pushee blindfolded. Begin slowly and develop intensity as confidence grows. You have to learn to "let go" with these drills and trust you body - much like the fabled blind man falling out of the cart. I wouldn't know about that myself of course... I've never been in a cart.

You can add in all the weapons work, disarms and so on into this as well. Also try having all parties blindfolded, though we suggest a sighted person be on hand to supervise. Try grappling, striking or just moving around.

Now let's try some psychological exercises. PA stands behind PB who is blindfolded. PA has a knife and slowly "stabs" with strong intent into PB's back. PB waits for the contact and moves away from the stab as per our usual drill. After a time, PB tries to move before contact. Not randomly but by "feeling" where the blade is coming. This all sounds a but "jedi" until people try it and begin to listen to their bodies. We rely on our sight an awful lot and that often screens out other ways in which we get information. Sometimes you will hear the person as they step, maybe feel their breath or smell them! If you "listen" enough you will also feel signal from your body. A slight twitch in a muscle, for example. Learn to listen to it, your body is trying to tell you something.

Once people have the feel, you can experiment with different object, increase the range, have both parties moving and so on. Be scrupulous and thorough when assessing results and don't kid yourself you are developing "superhuman" powers. This is a natural part of our make-up as any hunter will tell you!

From a close threat, we move out to something further away. This exercise needs a fair size space, we usually work it outdoors, especially at our camps as part of the low light training. The group splits into pairs. It is important that each pair works a distance away from each other to avoid interference.

The set up is this. PA assumes a position - standing, sitting or laying down. They are blindfolded. PB waits a fair distance away, then begins to slowly move towards PB, keeping their attention focused on their partner. When and if PA thinks they know where PB is they point to that place. PB immediately stops and PA removes the blindfold to see if they are correct. Once again, learn to use your full range of senses in order to pick up PB's approach. Try in different conditions and surroundings.

For more active awareness work you can try camouflage and concealment drills. On a basic level have one or more people hide and the rest look for them - hide and seek! You can add in all sorts of layers, depending on circumstances and surroundings. Give the hiders time to construct some camo, be it a few branches, a hide or a ghillie suit!

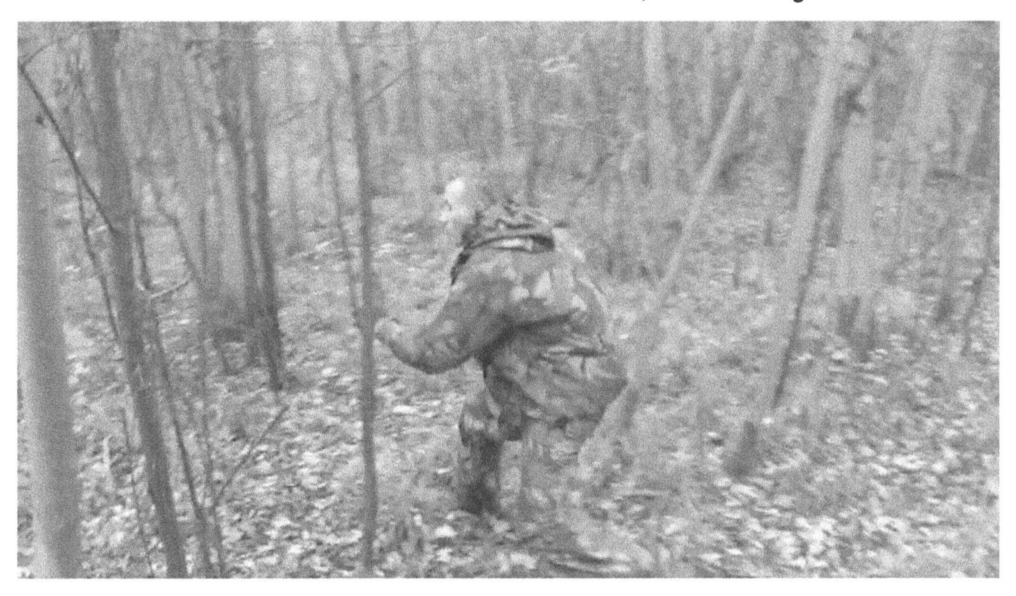

Having said that, when we talk of C&C most people assume a woodland setting. In fact you should be able to blend in anywhere. If it is safe to do so, have the group practice in an urban setting. The same rules of shape, shape, etc all still apply, but it is a different dynamic. If you want to add in "motivation" then give out tasks to be completed, even something as simple as moving from A to B. Please be aware of local sensitivities and any security issues!

Let's return to our regular training for one final psychological drill. We work in groups of four. PA is blindfolded. In turn, each of the rest of the group approach, place a hand on PA's shoulder and state their name. Repeat for a few times. After this, when the hand is placed in the shoulder, no name is given. PA must name the hand. Of course, mix up the order, otherwise it is very easy!

Being blindfolded in itself bring s a certain amount of fear and tension into the body. So let's now look at some drills designed to help us deal with those things. I want to stress very much here that dealing with fear, that is truly dealing with fear, is not about "toughing it out". It is about a balanced approach, which first recognises that we have and suffer from fear. Ignorance is not bliss and tough tends to become brittle.

Stage one is purely to experience some fear and begin using the breathing exercises to learn to cope. Fortunately, with the right friends around to help, fear and pain are never far away!

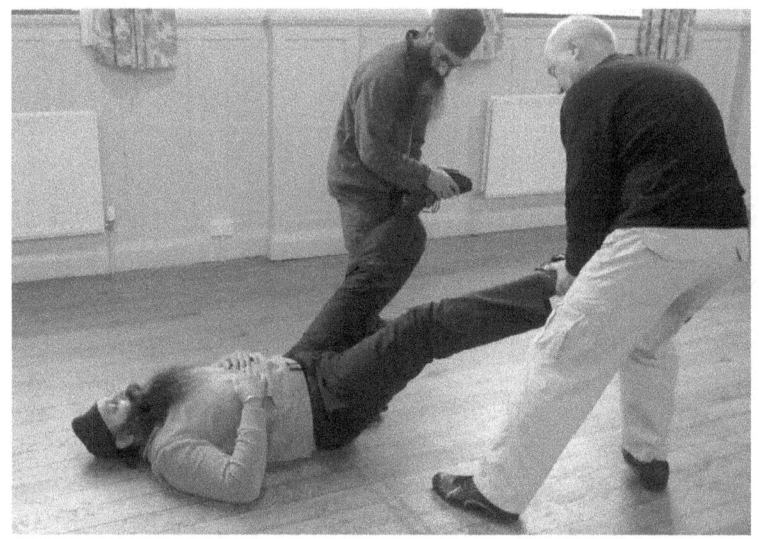

We previously described a drill where the arms and legs are twisted in order to help relax the muscles. We will return to that drill but with a twist - literally. PA lays on the floor and one or more partners twists their joints - wrists, ankles, fingers, etc.

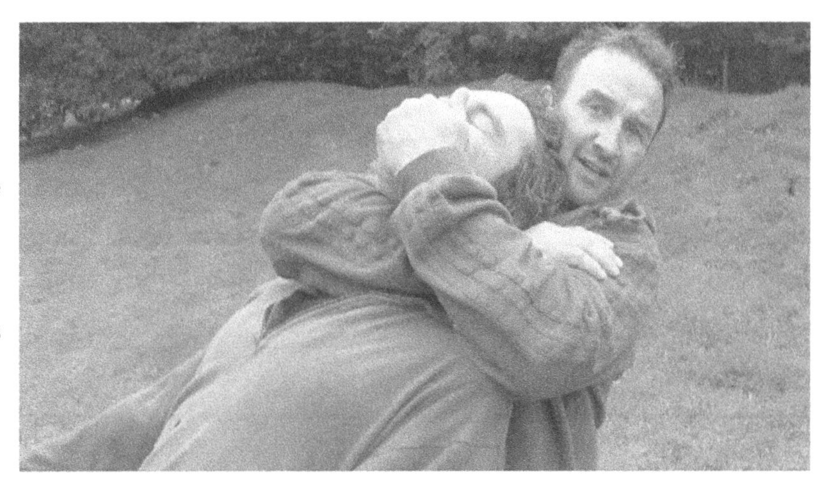

The twisters work slow but to the limit. PA uses breathing to relax into the fear and pain and manage it.

For the full experience there should be a person on each limb and another person administering helpful slaps, punches and pinches. But build up to that!

If you are working with trusted partners, then breath control is another rich area of fear training. Once people are familiar with holding their own breath, have them give control over to another person. This calls for sensitivity of course, but also we should not be too kind and deprive our training partner of a true experience. Simply have PB seal PA's nose and mouth during a breath hold. It is up to PB release when they feel it is time to do so.

You can work along similar lines with applying chokes, though again only with suitably experienced people.

We can also use weapons to address the fear issue. This drill uses the knife but can easily be adapted to other weapons to. PA and PB stand about 12 feet apart. PA moves the knife in a fixed pattern, say a left to

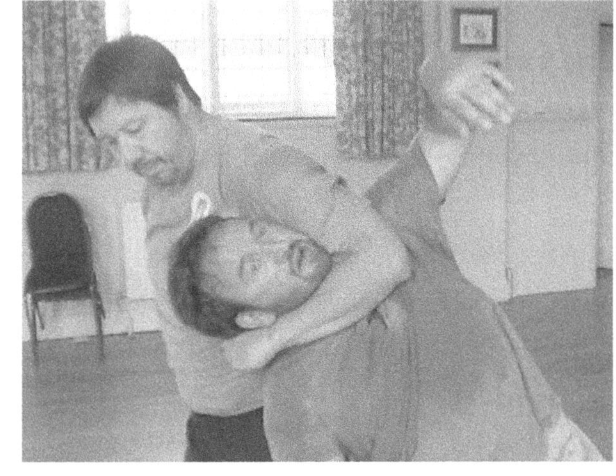

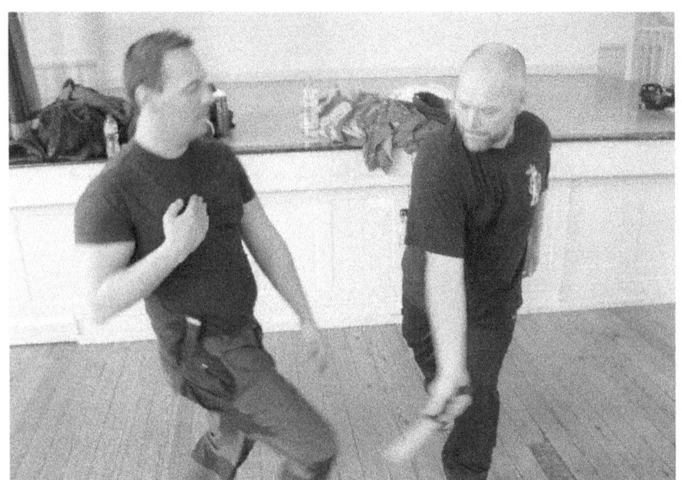

right slash. The movement should be reasonably slow and clear to start. PB has to walk to and past PA, avoiding contact with the knife but moving within touching distance of PA.

For the next stage, PB remains on the spot and PA walks towards them, waving the knife. PB avoids contact again. Finally, both partners walk towards each. It is important to note that PA is not trying to cut PB, they are just working a set movement. The pattern should change every few times and the speed increase. PB makes no move to disarm or touch PA for now, this is a fear drill, not a tactical one.

You can easily adapt this drill to work in groups, have two knife wielders for example, or work the gauntlet drills in this way.

If you prefer something more physical, try this next drill. This is partly about fear but also about working through pain. PA performs a set amount of the core exercises. A single partner or two or three others punch, slap and kick PA as they do the exercise. PA must use breathing to work through. Contact levels and reps can vary according to experience

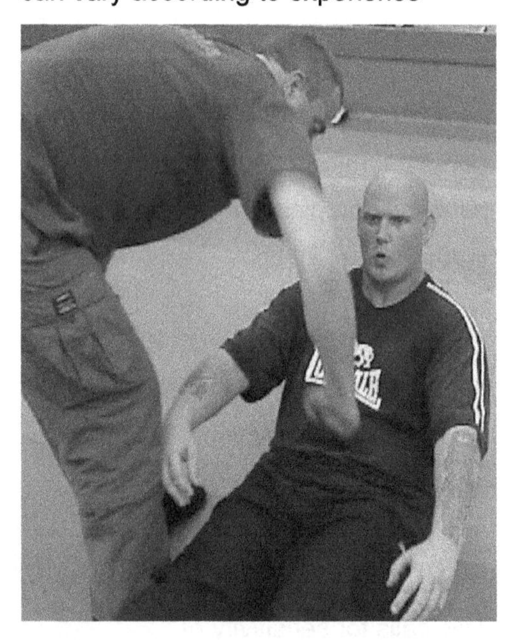

Let's now look at one of the Four Pillars with a range of exercises designed to develop good movement . We have already covered some ideas with gauntlet and zombie drills, let's look at the next level.

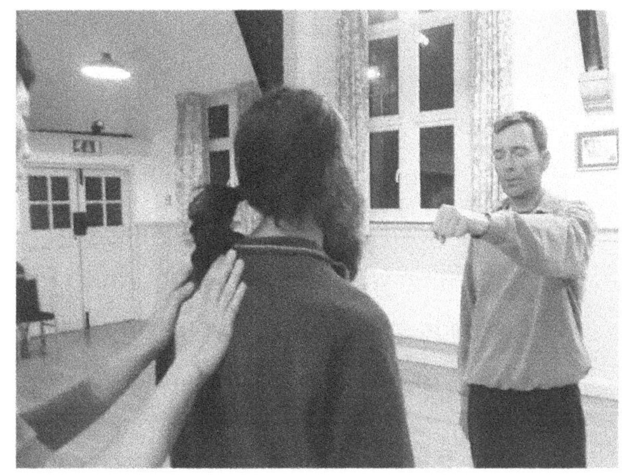

This is a three person drill. PA and PB face each other, about six feet apart. PC stands behind PA, PB extends a fist. PC gives PA a strong push towards PB. PA accepts the push and has to avoid the fist.

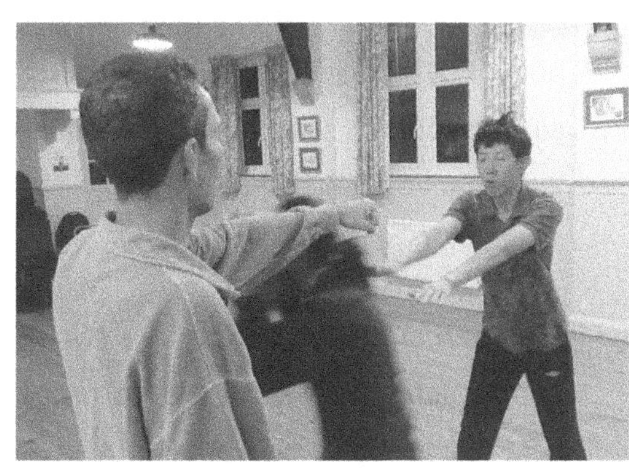

Run through a few times, then shorten the gap between PA and PB. Continue to shorten until the gap is about a foot. PC should give a decent shove. We find it also helps if PC closes their eyes - this avoids them moving the fist aside to protect PA!

You can add some other things into this drill too. Have PA start with hands down, as they are pushed forward they bring the hands up to protect the head and be ready to strike. As they dodge around PC, they can also carry out a takedown or strike. You can also make this a continuous drill. PA dodges around PC, then immediately turns and pushes them towards PB, who outstretches a fist.

One final variation is for PC not to extend the fist (or foot) until PA has been pushed, this obviously cuts down PA's reaction time even more.

If you have the space, tennis balls are a good way to get people moving. Work in pairs or a group. One person/s act as target, the others imply throw tennis balls at them, which the targets try to avoid.

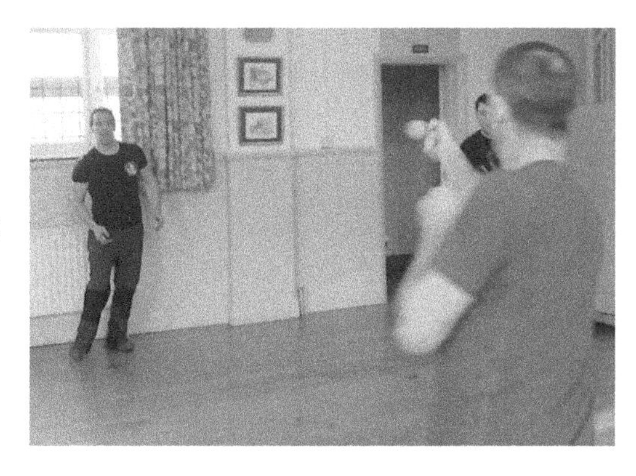

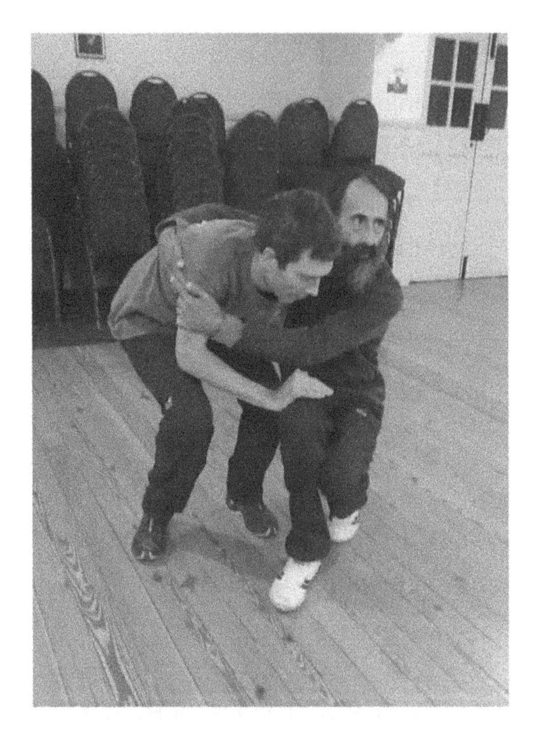

Grab and escape drills are another good method. PA tries to grab PB, who avoids the movement. There are a few variations to add in. PB can respond sooner or later. Sometimes it is useful to allow PA to contact, then move just before the hold is put fully on. After all you may not always see an attacker coming, anyone can get caught by surprise. PA can try different holds.

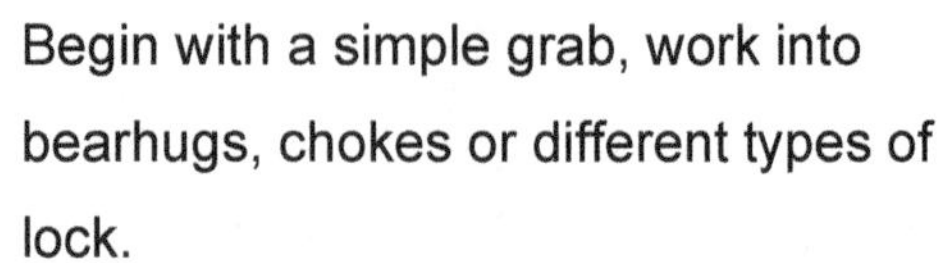

Begin with a simple grab, work into bearhugs, chokes or different types of lock.

You can turn this into a flow drill by having PA escape, then immediately repsond with their won grab, which PB avoids and so on. Or work two onto one or a free for all in a group.

If you want to work more on grab escapes, have PA apply a full grab or lock to PB. Once the hold is on, PB attempts to escape the hold through movement alone. First off, look to see what parts of the body you are able to move. Then see how you can affect PA's structure with that part of the body. For example, if you arms are pinned you can still move the hips and legs. So you could perhaps step around PA and work a hip throw.

For a bigger challenge have two people apply the hold. Again, allow the hold to come on then work to free yourself. When working against two, try as much as you can to join them together. You can often use one to off-balance or impede the other.

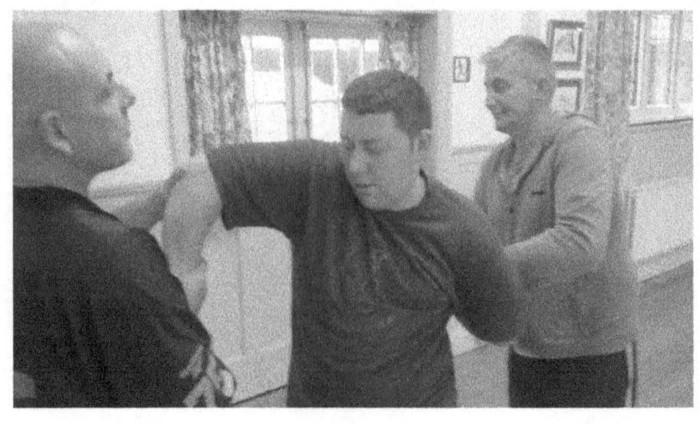

For the moving version of this last drill, simply have two people grab your wrist and try and lock your arm. You can use soft movement or selective tension to prevent this, also once again try and join the two people together.

If you want to work on maintaining posture while in movement, try this. PA places a hand on the back of PB's head. Using light pressure they then move PB around the room. PA's job is imply to respond to direction changes as smoothly as possible, whilst maintaining good posture. It is important that the hips remain relaxed and the footwork light and agile. For extra work, add in level changes too. You can experiment with using different parts of the body to lead the movement. This is important as you should not rely on one part of the body to always initiate movement. If something is thrown at your face, it is natural to move the head first. If you get "stuck" in the feet, your response will be slowed.

You can work with this notion of hand leading movement by trying this exercise. PA walks towards PB and "flows" around them - ie avoid contact but keep close. When you get near to PB, point your hand towards the space you are moving into. The rest of your body follows this hand movement.

Now PA stands still and PB moves towards them, with some kind of threatening posture. PA once again "points" the hand into the relevant space and the body moves into it. Once you have the idea with the hand, use the foot or other part.

Then return to the hand. You can of course increase speed or add in more people. When the hand points now, it should also make light contact as the body moves through. This helps develop precision and accuracy in hand placement while on the move, whether for takedowns or strikes, both of which you can finally add in.

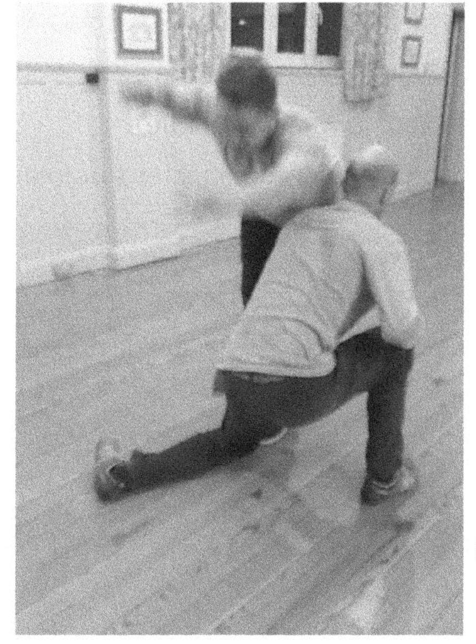

S

For a slightly different version of this exercise, have a group stand quite close together. PA must now move through the group as smoothly as possible. Experiment again with using the hand to find the space then lead the body into it. For extra challenge, have the group link arms and/or close in tight and see how PA can work through the gaps.

We have mentioned sensitivity a few times already and working with a partner is a great way to develop tactile awareness and response. The simplest method is to use the sticky hands type drills we mentioned before and have one partner follow the others movement. From here we can branch off into many variations. Contact with different parts of the body, such as we did during the partner core exercises. You can go with fixed or free movement and work in threes or fours.

Another thing to try is not to be in direct physical contact but to have an object in between.

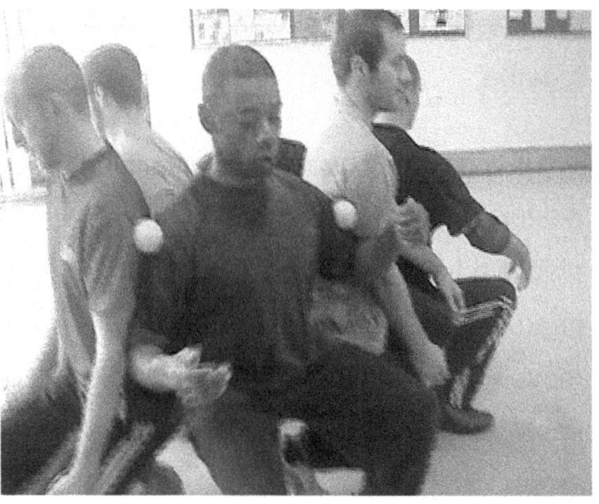

As an example, try the Core Exercises in pairs of more, but with a tennis ball between each person. This calls for a different degree of sensitivity, plus also the idea of "communication" through an object.

You can work in a similar way, with any size ball and make the movement more freeform. For example give the pair or group a specific task or course to follow. Start with a simple straight line, then add in level changes and different types of obstacle. The aim is always to keep movement as fluid as possible.

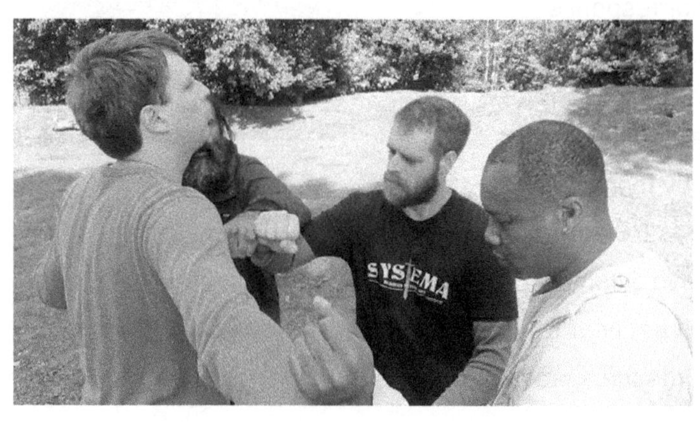

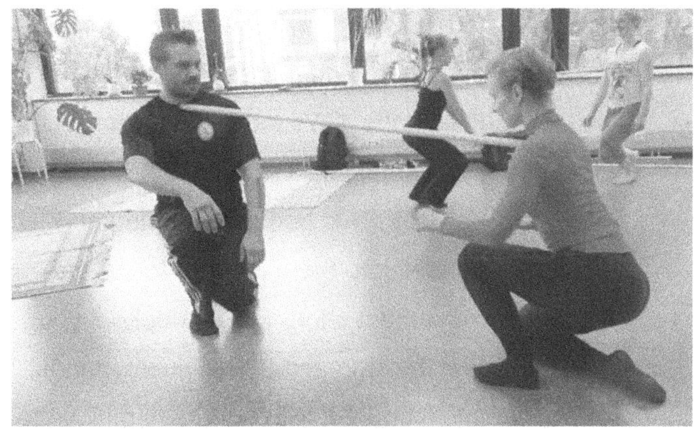

other and grasp each others arms. Each raises a leg and makes contact with it. Both partners now simply moves the leg around whilst maintaining contact. The holding is to help you keep balance, but after a while you should work from free standing.

Once you have the idea, PA can work to kick the PB's supporting leg or a similar attacking move while PB defends (from contact). Switch roles, then both attack and defend simultaneously. If one person is not sure of their balance, you can do the same drill but use a stick to contact the leg. PA simply has to stay in contact with the stick.

We can work in a similar way with sticks. Being in pairs, PA and PB face each other with a stick in-between. The stick rests on the body, do not hold it with the hands. Partners begin to move and must not let the stick drop. Once again, simple moves at first, then level changes and more challenging movements.

Repeat the same, with three or four people. This again calls for another level of sensitivity.

So we have covered sensitivity with the arms and the body, how about the legs? Well, we can work "sticky leg" drills with the following set up. PA and PB stand facing each

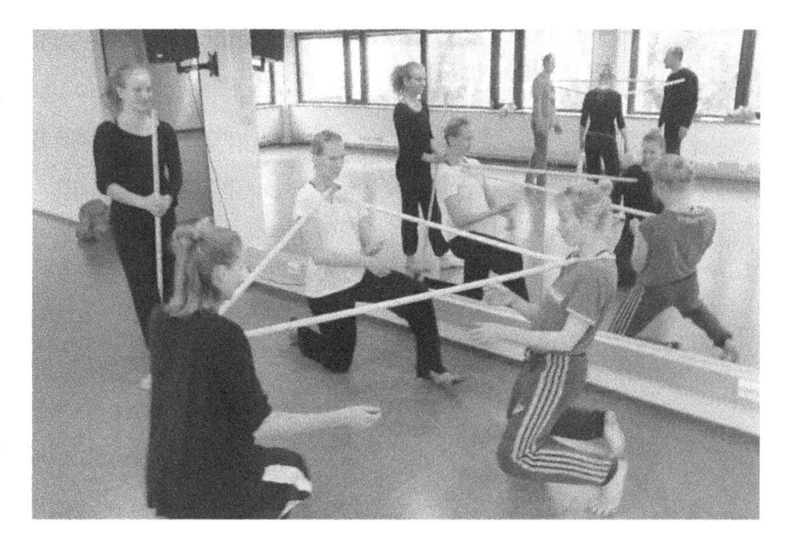

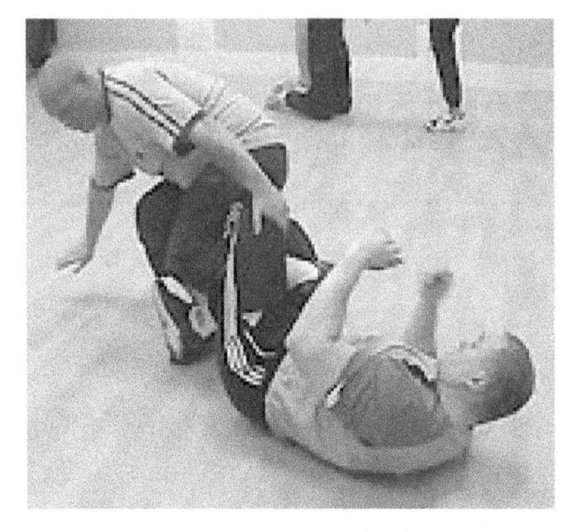

For a groundwork version, PA lays on the floor and PB approaches. This can be a simple walk, a stamp or kick or grappling attack. PA is only allowed to use their legs to deflect or move away PB.

While we are on the floor , let's look at one more sensitivity drill. This teaches us about felling and working with tension and can be translated into stand up work too. PA lays on their back, PB kneels over them and places their hands on PA's body. PA's job is simply to get up, slowly at first. PB has to feel which parts of PA's body are tensing and pushes into them in order to cut the movement short. For example, if you feel the stomach tense, push your fist into it and PA will find it very difficult to move. PB can also watch for support -

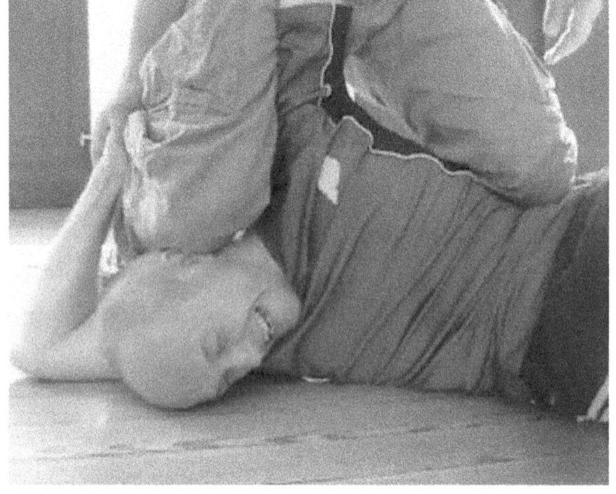

where PA places a hand on the floor to push up, sweep it away, for example. They can also use leverage - a little pressure on the forehead makes it difficult to sit up!

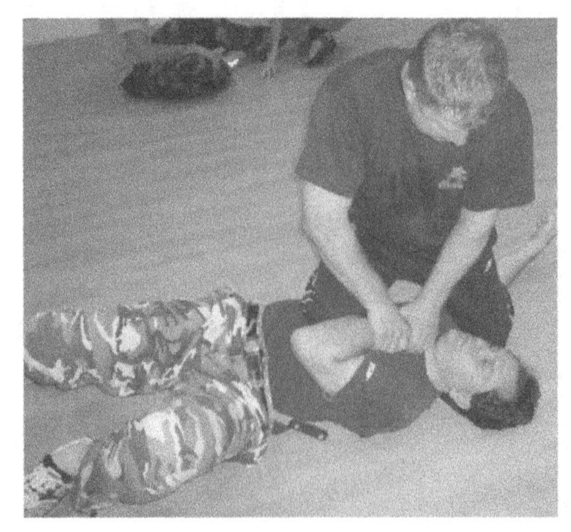

For PA this is an exercise in moving with minimal tension and working around obstacles. Following this, PB works by kneeling on PA for the same procedure. Finally, PB works standing and uses the feet for the same procedure. You can, of course, repeat with PA laying on their front too.

Balance is a big component of movement, so here are some ideas on developing balance with a partner. The most basic drill is for PA to stand and keep balance while PB pulls or pushes on different parts of the body. To increase the challenge, PA stands on one leg. You can also work this in groups of three or more

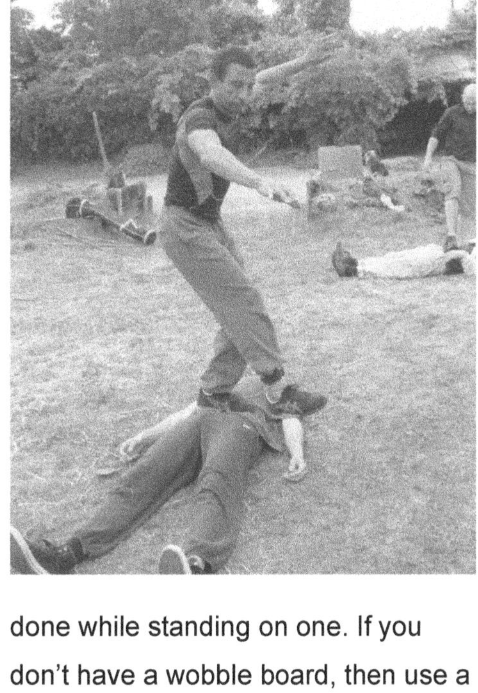

If in a group, have PA stand in the middle of a circle of four people. They then lift a foot and must push/kick each person in the group at least once without putting the foot back down on the floor.

Wobble boards are useful addition to this type of work, you can carry out the above or many other drills we have done while standing on one. If you don't have a wobble board, then use a friend! Stand on them, front/back and perform movements are be pushed and pulled by another person as above.

You can simply increase the challenge level of any balance exercise by having the person close their eyes too, as this has a negative effect on our balance.

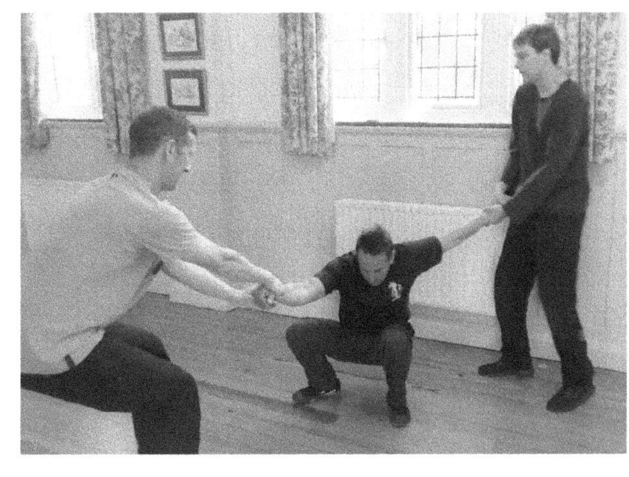

To work in a more dynamic way, simply take any of the sensitivity exercises we did earlier and try them on one leg - either one partner at a

time, or both / all. Try not to lean too much on your partner when doing so, as support can be quickly taken away!

Some of earlier drills touched on reaction time. Let's look at that in a little more detail. The first step to developing good reactions is awareness - if you don't know it's there you can't react to it! The second step is for the body to be relaxed in order that it can move as swiftly as possible. Remember, smooth is fast!

We have covered tactile awareness and intuition, so we will take a look at a couple of drills to develop hand/eye co-ordination. We go back to using the tennis ball for the first. PA stands behind PB and throws the ball over PB's shoulder. This should be an up throw, so the ball describes a large arc over the shoulder. As soon as PB sees the ball they should catch it. Begin with a three count, as we did with the knife drop exercise. Then go to a one count, then no count at all. You can decrease the distance / arc of the throw for a greater challenge.

The next drills work off of picking up another person's movement. The first version is for PA and PB to stand facing each other. PA makes some movement, it should be quite large at first. As soon as they see the movement, PB points to it and exhales. PB should learn to scan the whole body with "soft vision" rather than have tunnel vision on just a hand or foot.

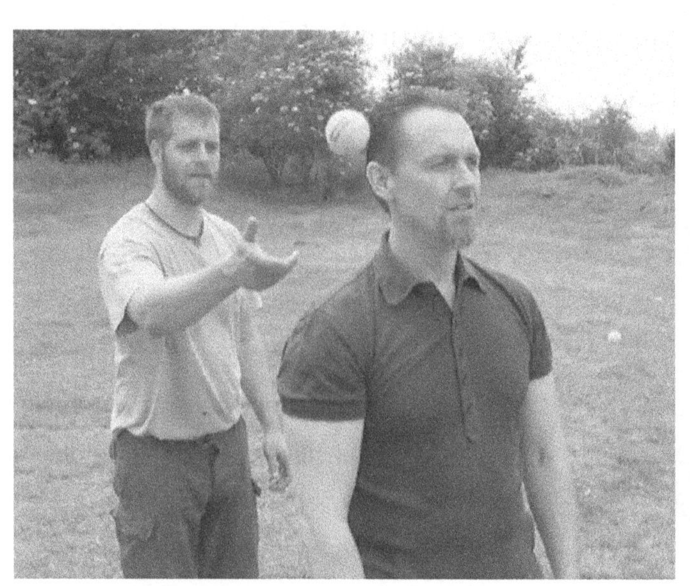

Following this, PA makes smaller movements, down to even just tensing a specific muscle group. You can repeat with PA facing two or more people for a greater challenge.

For our final exercise, partners sit

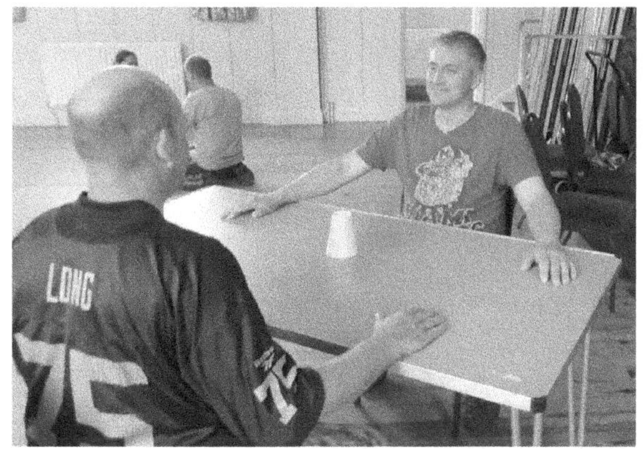

opposite each other at a table. Place an object in between, within reach of both people. We suggest a plastic cup or similar, something non-sharp and non-breakable. The aim is simple - be the first to grab the cup!

To conclude this section I just wanted to mention one more aspect of "partner training" which develops all sorts of attributes and that is working with animals. Horse riding develops a wealth of skills, from tactile sensitivity to communication to good posture and fear control! With a little thought and imagination it is possible to work many partner and group drills in with horses too.

Finally, there is working with dogs. We are fortunate to have colleagues who run a large security organisation, including K9 work. Once again, the development

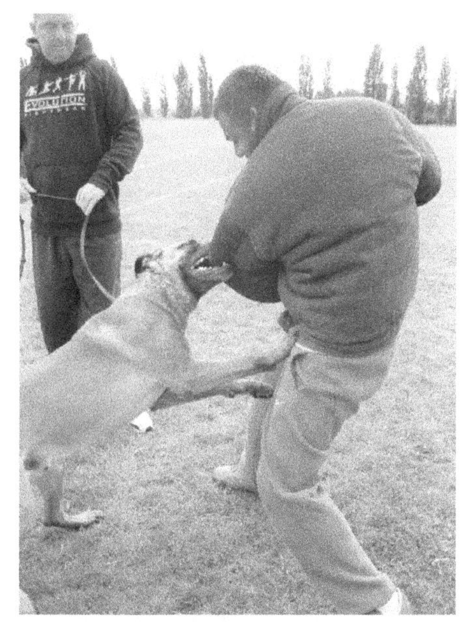

of communication between human and animal is fascinating and the chance to undergo the attack training from the bad-guy end is very educational for fear control!

Both of these obviously call for expert instruction but I mention them as food for thought!

CHAPTER TEN
MASSAGE

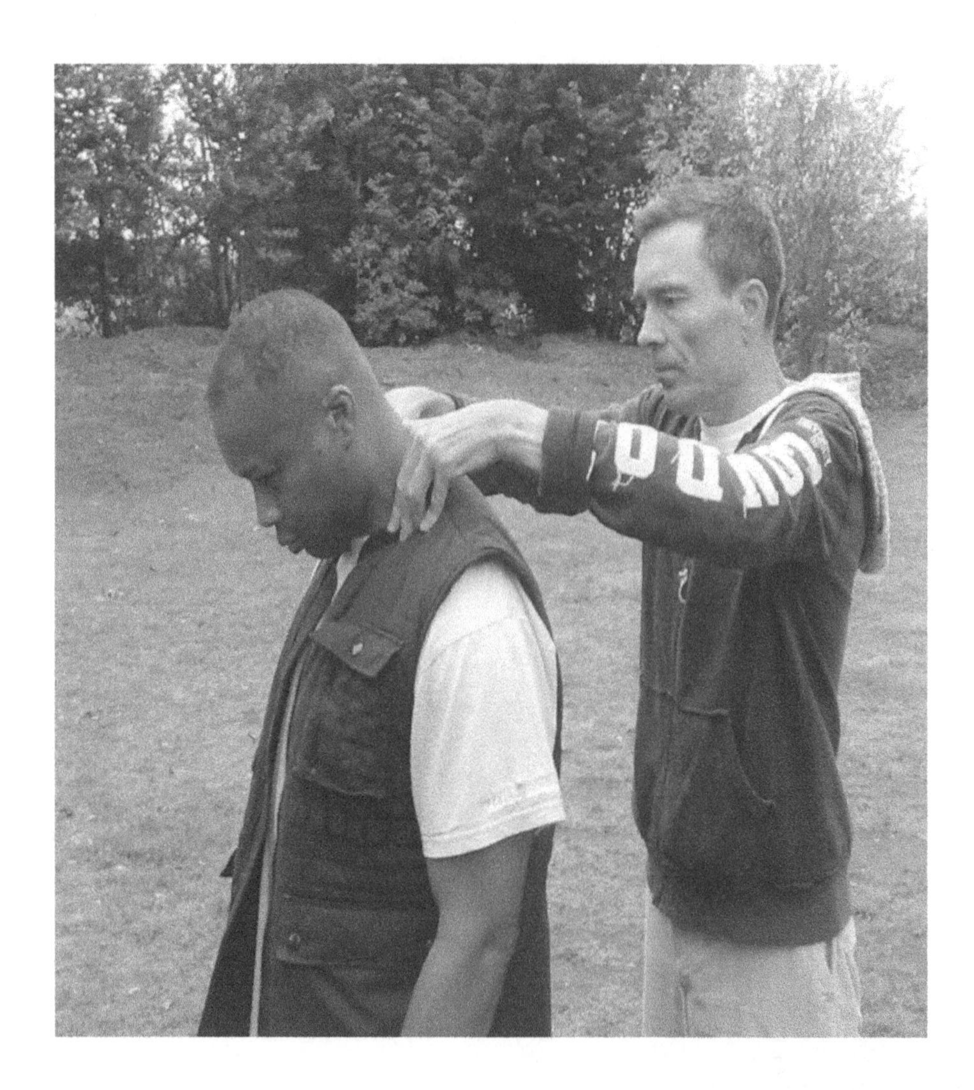

MASSAGE

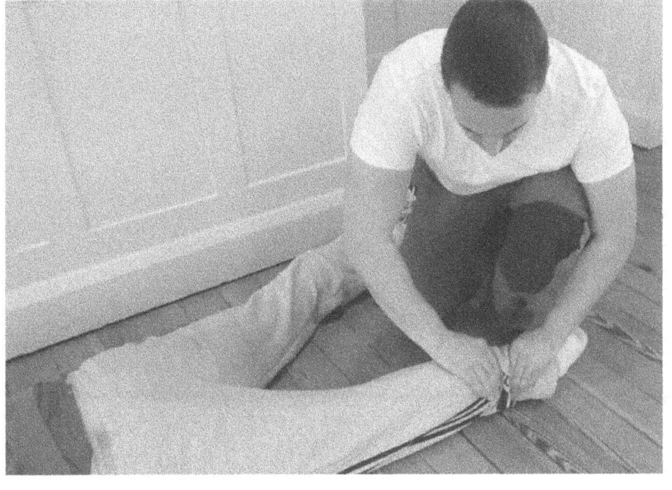

We know that health training is an important aspect of Systema training, in fact it is the most important. A primary concern of any of our training methods, whatever their purpose, is that they are non-destructive to the practitioner. In our previous book we covered some ideas on diet and general well-being as well as specific self massage ideas. Obviously, with a partner we have far more scope for massage.

As with our earlier stretching, the goal of massage is to encourage relaxation within the body, to rid ourselves of unnecessary tension. That tension may be on the surface, it may be the result of bumps taken in training, or it may lay much deeper within and be linked into emotional issues or past injuries or traumas. This means that massage can also be a powerful tool for dealing with our problems on a wide and deep level.

Do not be surprised if unlocking a person's physical tension also unlocks some emotional tension. This is quite normal and should not be either discouraged nor sought for. Simply let the work do its work.

Once again, if you are massaging a person you should ask if they have any medical or other issues and work accordingly. If in doubt, always refer to a healthcare professional. Be sensitive to your partner. Some massage is immediately painful but longer term beneficial. Do not be too "kind" but neither should you see yourself as an inflicting punishment and "no pain no gain" on your partners.

Keep your ego in check too. I've seen people rush to help anyone with back ache or a stiff shoulder, sometimes in inappropriate times or places, in a bid to be seen as a great healer. Never give massage where it is not wanted and

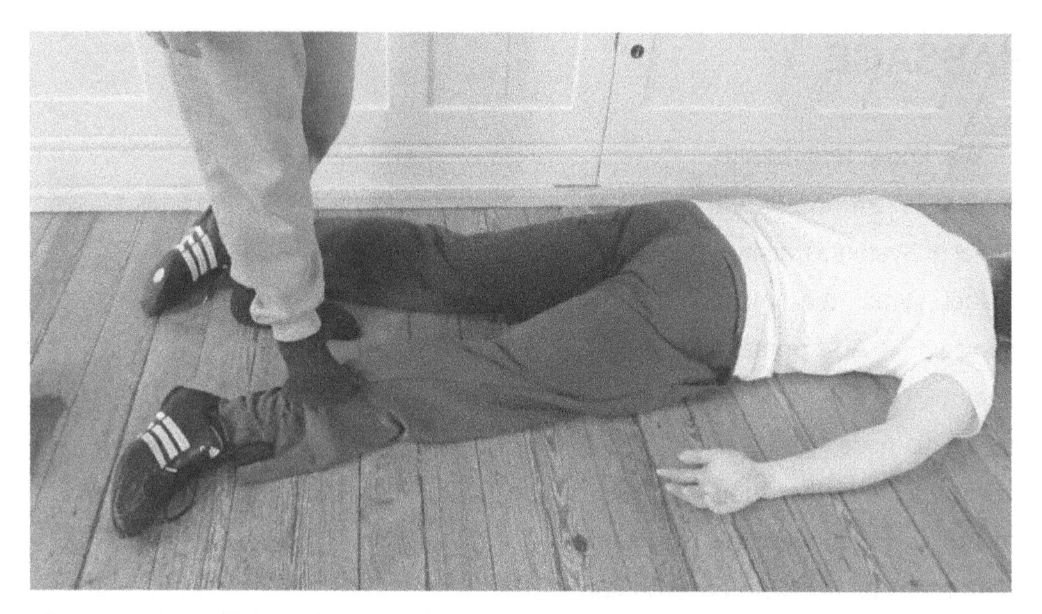

always start light if people are inexperienced. Even a light touch can bring psychological discomfort, so please be aware. If you want to take your studies further, their is a huge amount of information and course available in many different types of bodywork, at least study the basics of anatomy.

We are covering the basic massage methods here. These are the ones we use most often in class, either at the start as preparation, or at the end of the class to eases out any strains or knots. Sometimes both! It is good to feature some kind of massage of manipulation work in every class if you can, it brings so many benefits. Time spent depends on how much time you have, but for a quick basic massage you need to allow at least five minutes per person.

It is good to have somewhere warm and reasonably comfortable, but we have done massage outdoors in all types of situation to. As with all the work, this is for life, not just the training room.

For the person being massaged, all you have to do is relax and breathe. Listen to instructions, if there are any and try and let the massage penetrate deep into your muscles. Where there is particular tension, you can try the breath-hold tense, exhale release protocol we worked in stretching. If you have any concerns, relay them to your partner. If things get too intense, ask to stop. There can be a certain amount of discomfort involved but it should never be more than you can handle

THE BACK WALK

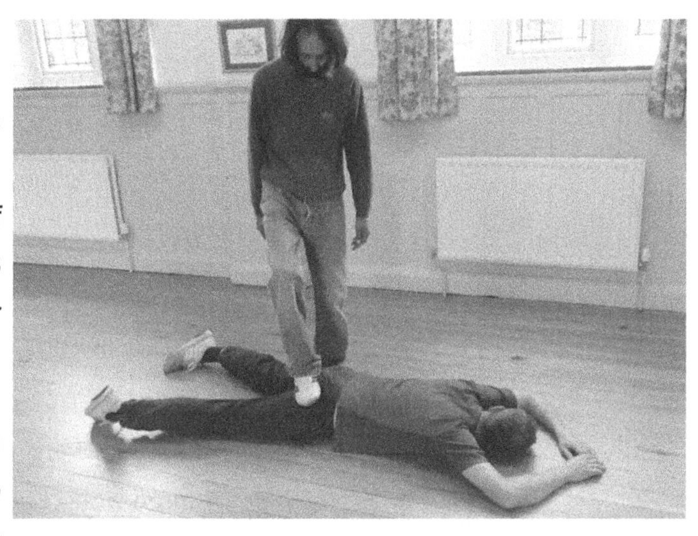

PA lays face down in the floor, PB is standing. Both are barefoot, if practical. If required, PB can use a stick, chair or wall for support.

PB begins by using their foot to work into PA's feet. Push into the arches with a squeezing motion, a bit like you are pressing down on a brake pedal. Work both feet for an equal amount of time.

PA turns one foot out to the side, so the knee is pointing outwards. PB now begins to work along the calf with their foot, squeezing down as before, working up and down the muscle. Never put weight on the rear of the knee.

Once both calves are done, PA returns the legs to their original position. PB now begins to walk up and down the thighs – individually or both together. Once again, take care not to step on the rear of the knees.

PB works up to the butt, then turns one foot out ninety degrees and places

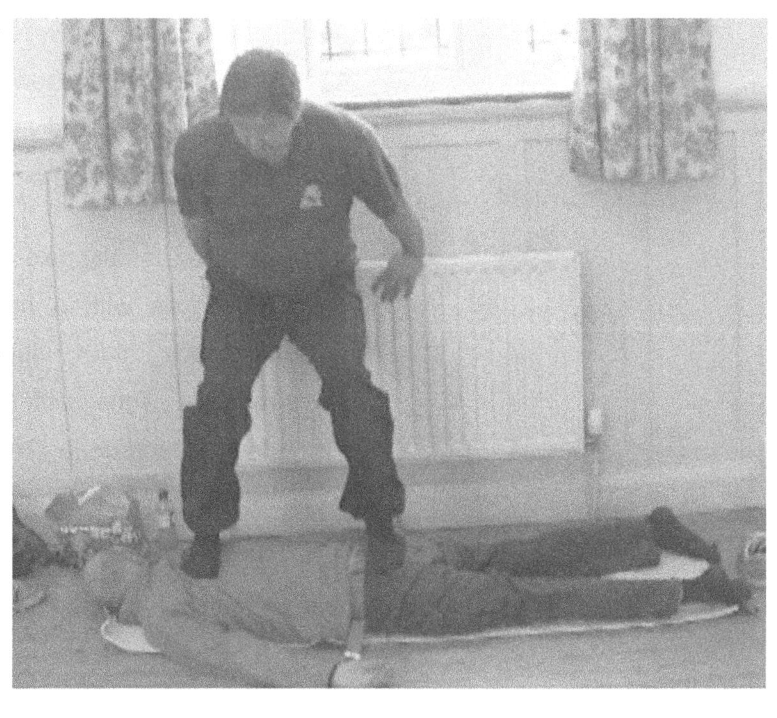

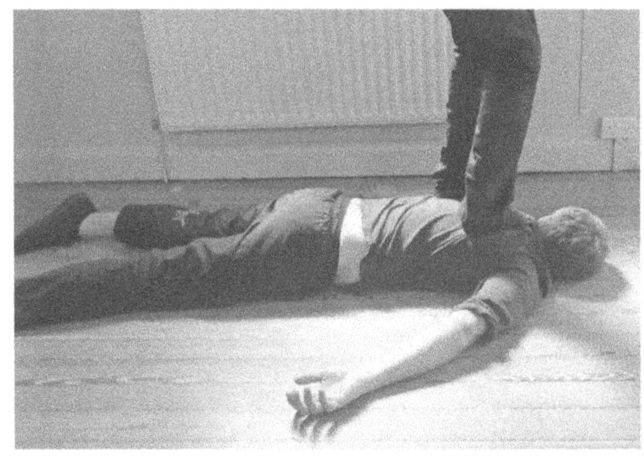

it on the lower back, just about the coccyx. Never put direct weight on the kidneys. The other foot, also turned out to ninety degrees, begins to slowly walk up and down the spine, easing the weight into it as before. Work across the spine and never along it. Go up and down a few times, you may hear some clicks, this is fine. Remember, take care in the kidney area.

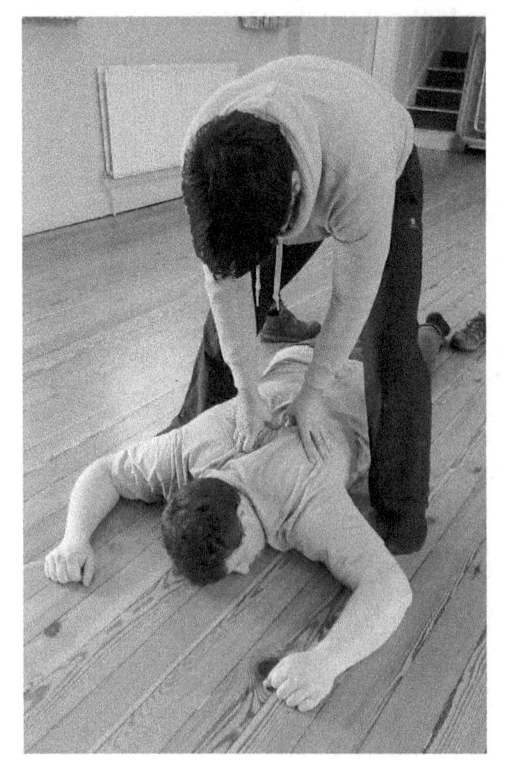

Once you have walked the spine, you can use one or both feet to work the shoulder area. Try to feel where there is most tension and give those areas more work. Feet are very sensitive and more mobile than we might think, so learn to use your whole foot to deliver the massage.

Once done, slowly move your feet out to the tops of the arms. You can keep a heel on the floor or put the full weight on the arms, working into the muscles again. Work down, avoiding direct pressure on the elbow, to the hands. PA turns palms up and you use your toes to massage into the hands.

We usually like to conclude the procedure with a coupe of assisted stretches, then vigorously rub the muscles of the back from the shoulder down. Once done, PA should rest for a moment before getting up slowly.

You can also repeat this method on the front, ie PA lays on their back. Be aware again that you are not putting direct pressure on soft areas, work into the muscles.

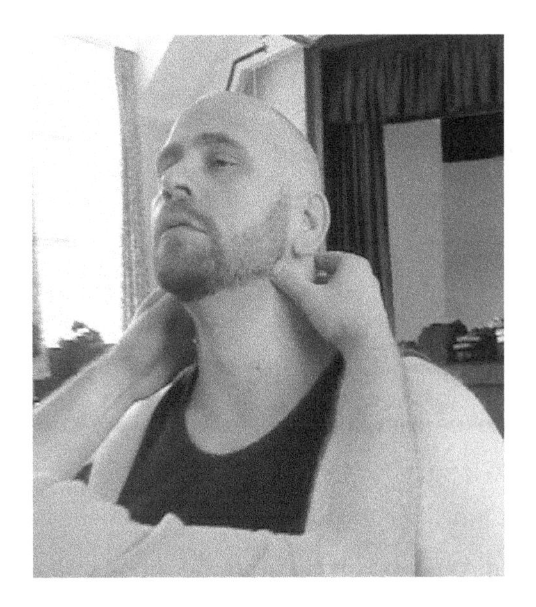

OTHER MASSAGES

There are several ways of delivering a massage. They include stroking, kneading, pushing, twisting, percussive, using heat and more. The most basic form is to knead the muscles like dough. Have your partner sit, stand behind them with hands on shoulders and work into the muscles around the shoulders and neck. This can be light at first, becoming more vigorous as required. You will find massage develops good hand strength too! This simple method can be used for all the major muscle groups

HEAD

Let's work through a head and neck massage that illustrates a few different ways of working. PA sits, PB stands behind and rests their hands on PA's shoulders. Both breath and relax. PB now rubs their hands together to develop some heat, then places one palm on the base of the skull, the other on the crown of the head. Let the hands be relaxed and heavy, imagine passing the heat between your palms. Now move one palm up to the crown and the other to the centre of the forehead. Hold again for a couple of minutes.

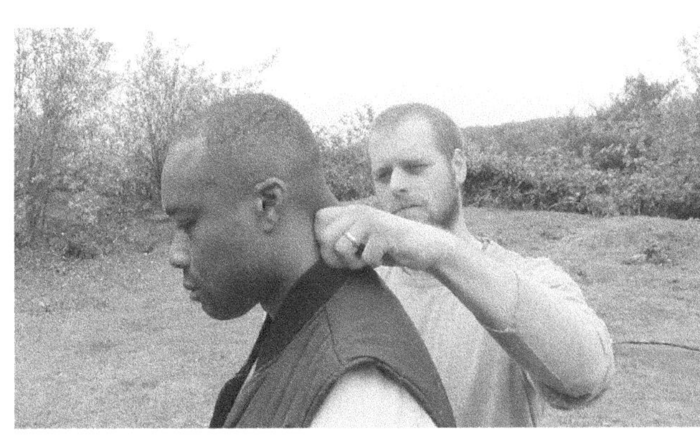

After this, using the fingertips, gently massage the area around PA's temple and eyes. Work into the hinge of the jaw, then gently around the ears. Now, using your fingertips, start at the crown of the head and begin tapping, working out

and down. Tap the fingers onto the skull, once you reach the lower part, return to the top and begin again. Cover the whole skull.

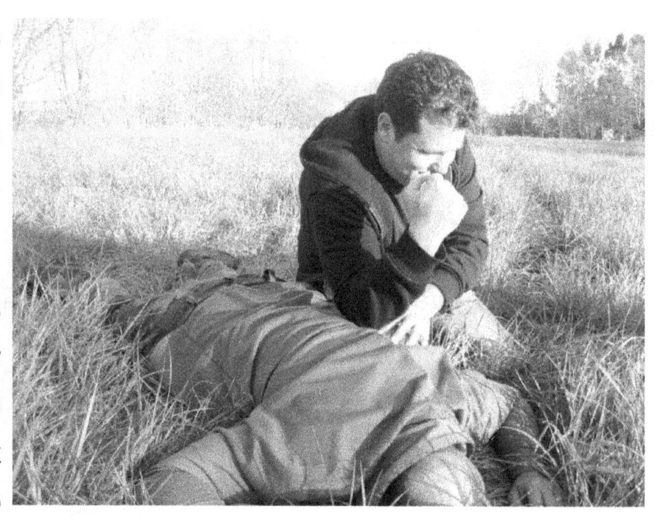

Following this, PA drops their chin forward. PB now strokes with fingertips down the long muscles on the back of the neck. If there is deep tension, work into it with the thumbs. If you wish you can add in a neck manipulation here, moving the head sharply to one side to "crack" the neck.

To finish, return to the start position with hands rested on shoulders. Both partners take a little time to breathe and relax again.

TRIGGER POINT

A trigger point is a tense spot in a muscle that causes pain in other parts of the body. It may be felt as a knot or hard spot in the muscle. TP massage involves simply pushing into the sore spot with isolated pressure. Use a thumb, knuckle or piece of equipment (see later). The recipient should inhale and tense as the push comes in. Hold for a little, with the pressure maintained, then burst breath. The basic idea is to overload the muscle with tension until it is forced to relax.

CALF STAND

This is a great method of dealing with tension in the legs, but it can be

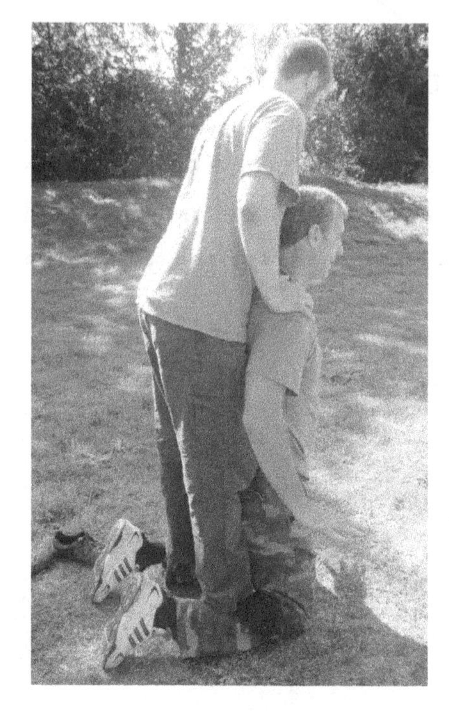

quite intense! PA kneels down - you may wish to put something soft under the knees. PB simple walks up and down the calves. You can work one at a time, or both together. Ease and squeeze the tension out, a bit like toothpaste from a tube!

FIST MASSAGE

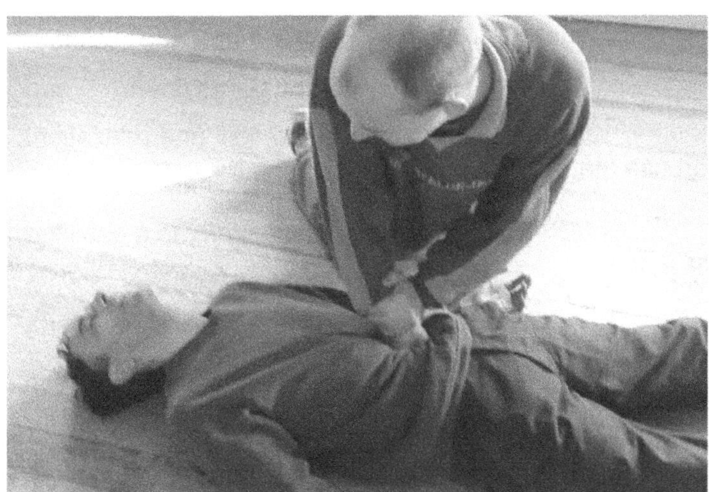

To work deeper into the organs, try this exercise. PA lays on the back. PB kneels and slowly pushes their fist into PA's abdomen. PA should try and relax completely. When the first tension barrier is met, pause and hold the push there. PA follows the "stretch protocol". On exhale, PB should be able to push in a little deeper.

Work all round the abdomen, then repeat with PA on their front.

USING TOOLS

As well as pushing the hands to massage, there are a variety of tools we can use. Some of them are specialist, such as the deer horns or various other devices. However it is easy to use some every objects to assist with massage.

Working with a stick is one. You can use it to roll along the muscle or to press into specific points. You can also use it to deliver strikes to the muscle too, in order to promote relaxation.

Once you have that idea, you will see how you can massage with almost anything. Even a knife can

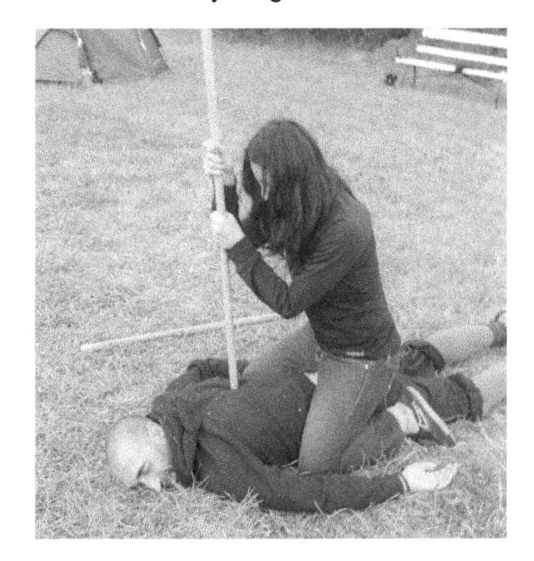

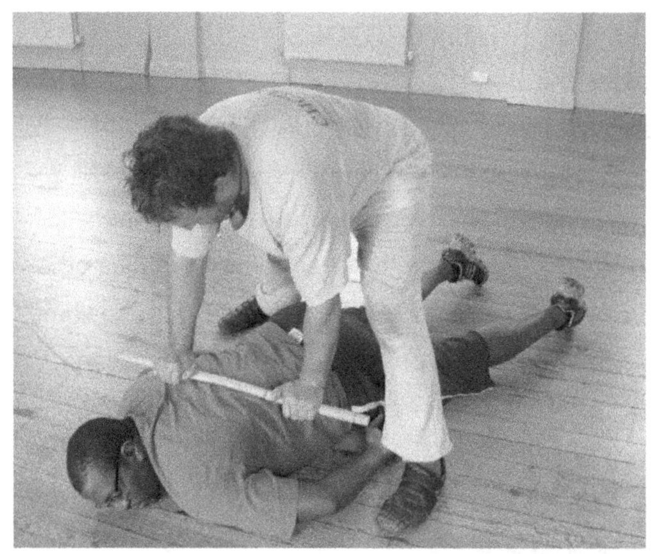

work well, see how you can use the hilt like a stick, the flat of the blade to stroke and even the point to some extent!

For rotation work, look at using a ball, foam roller, or a plastic bottle filled with warm water. One way to use that latter is place it under PA's back, then lift their feet and roll them back and forth so the bottle goes up and down their spine.

THE WHIP

The whip is a great tool for massage. There is nothing quite like it for waking up the central nervous system and encouraging blood flow and relaxation! We cover the basics here, for more in-depth work please refer to a qualified instructor.

PA stands or lays down. PB folds the whip and lightly brushes all round PA's muscles. This is to prepare the body for contact. Following this, keeping the

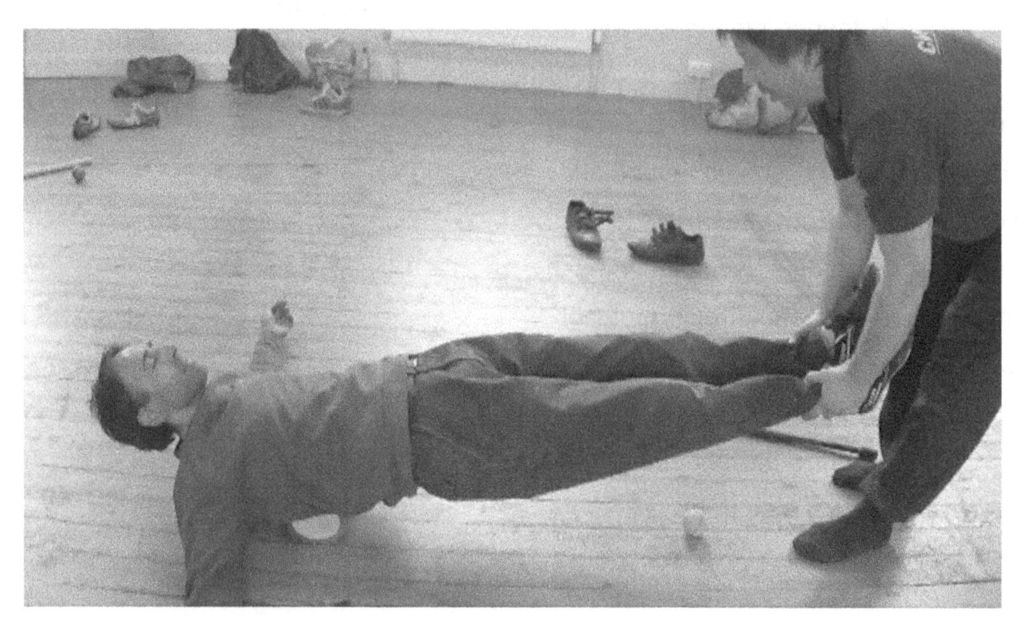

SYSTEMA PARTNER TRAINING

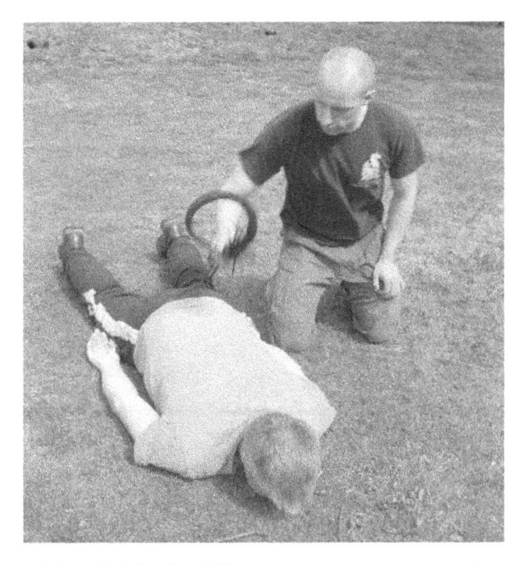

whip folded, PB begins tapping the muscles. Repeat with harder strikes.

After this, PB strikes into the muscles with the tip of the whip. Experiment with angles and depth of strike. Allow time to recover between each strike. A single strike on its own may be bearable, but a barrage of even light strikes can overwhelm the CNS.

Work all around the body, paying particular attention to the areas of greatest tension. Allow the recipient some "quiet time" to recover.

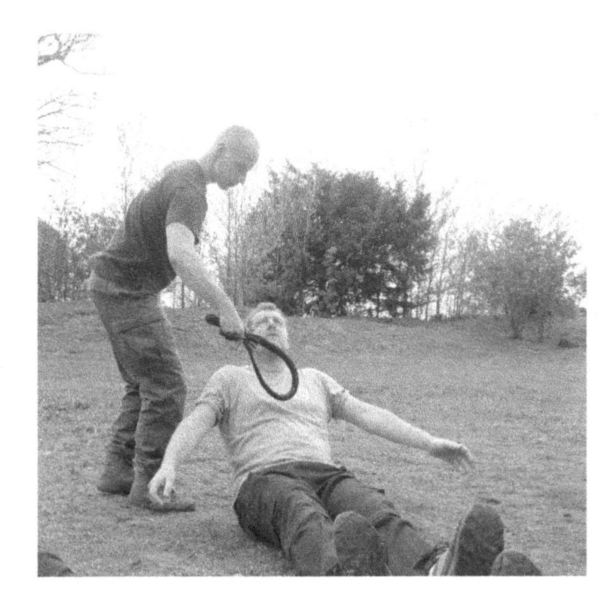

These are some of the basic types of massage, but they should suffice for most regular class work. For more advanced and specific types of work we refer you to the resources put out by Toronto HQ and others.

Of course, where possible, learn under the leading teachers too, they are a great source of information for this kind for work. Outside of that, as mentioned already, there are numerous other types of resources available for different types of massage. The key to this work is practice and sensitivity. Try and work massage into your daily routine, for yourself, for your family. It is probably our oldest form of healing and the therapeutic benefits of touch should not be ignored.

CHAPTER ELEVEN
CONCLUSIONS

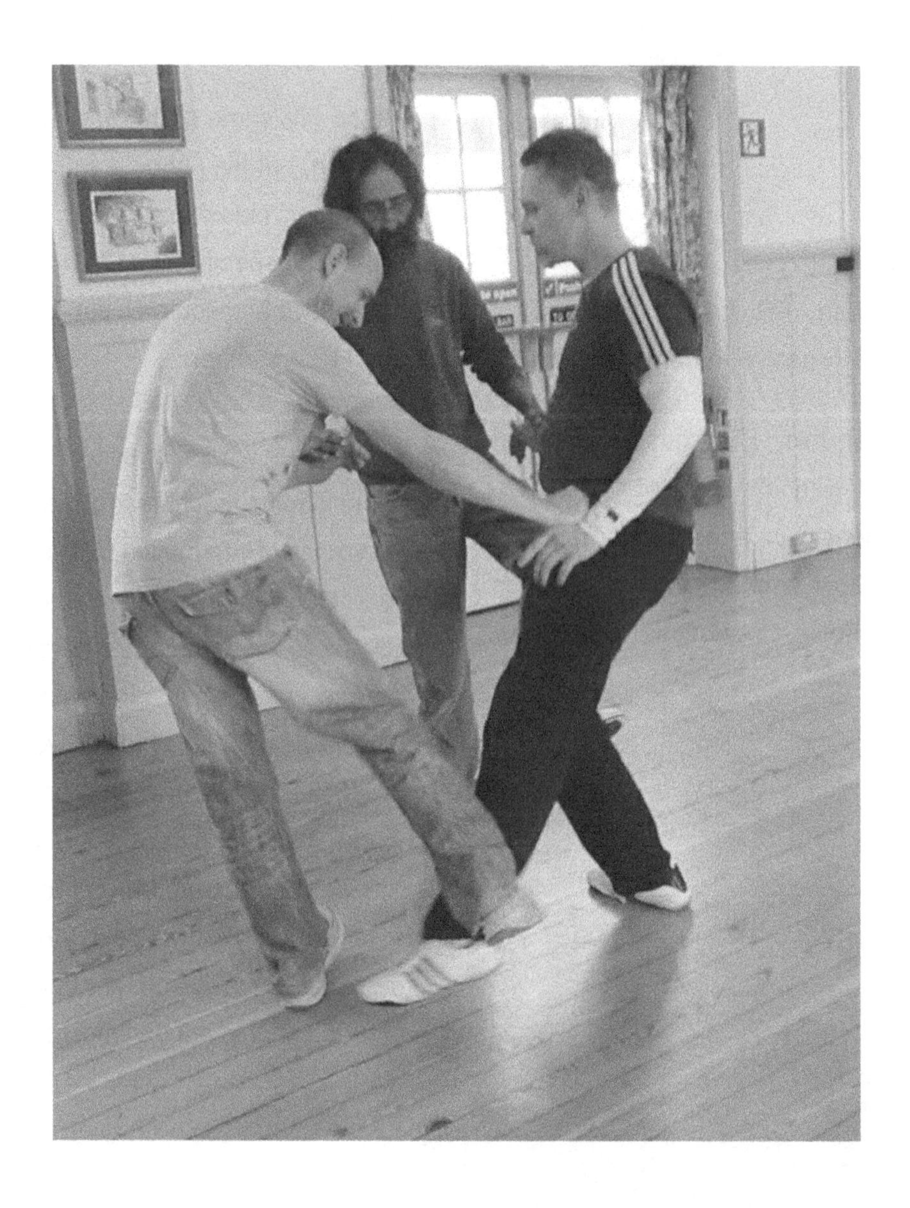

CONCLUSIONS

We've covered all the major areas of working with a partner and, I hope, given you a strong base from which to develop your own ideas. As mentioned at the start, it would be impossible to include every exercise type or variation in one book, so bear in mind that what you see here is just the start!

If you are lucky enough to have access to regular training partners I recommend choosing a few exercises at a time, perhaps by topic, and running through them. At the root of everything lay the Four Pillars, most especially breathing, so please be aware of their role in every exercise you do. Also be aware of the needs of your partner and help them to develop. By doing so, everyone in the group grows together.

Vary the intensity of your sessions too. Systema not about driving yourself hard into the ground at every available opportunity, nor is it about being "easy" on yourself. The aim is to get a good overall balance in your exercise regime. It is important to maintain balance in our training, so please don't over-emphasise one area at the expense of another. Work strength training with mobility, speed with relaxation, above all always deal with any extra stress brought into your system with breathing and massage. Always be sure to check with your healthcare professional prior to exercising if you have a medical condition and if any exercise causes you undue pain or distress, stop it immediately!

Please take on board what we have said about adapting and creating exercises for your own needs. There are also many other resources, many Systema Instructors and others put lots of good ideas out on social media, for example. Also please understand how "exercise" can actually be part of your everyday activities. If you can grasp

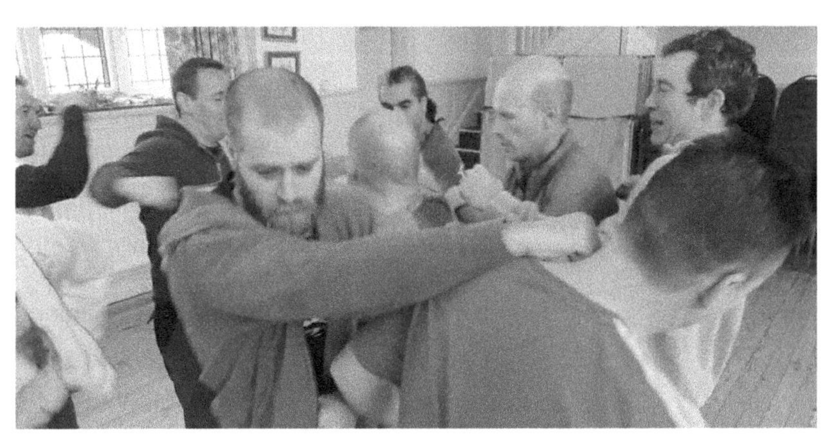

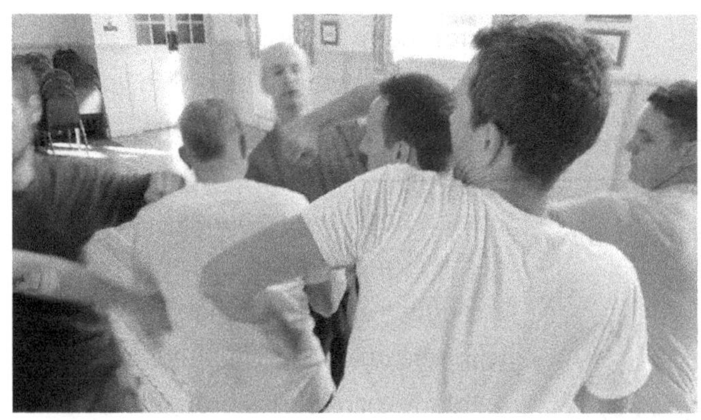

this, you can be training all the time, especially if you can get your family involved!

One very important aspect of group training is the Circle Up at the end of each training session. In case you do not already do this, I will describe it. The very last thing we do in class is sit in a circle and, starting at one end, everyone has the opportunity to share some thoughts about what has gone before. This can be a simple "liked this, didn't like that" or it can go further, depending on time constraints.

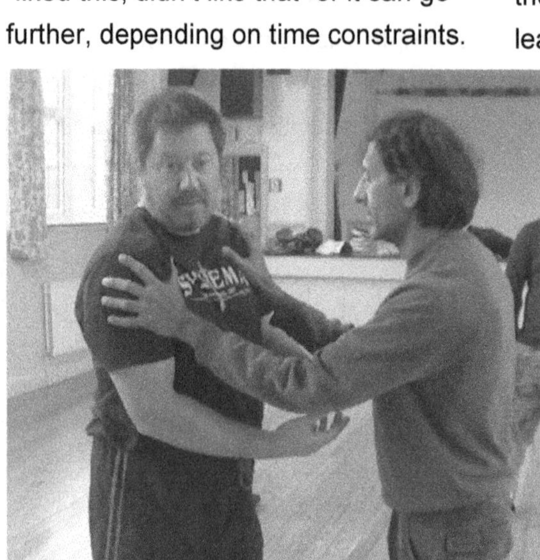

The important thing is that everyone has a voice and input. Over the years I have found this to be a unique, useful and sometimes extremely profound experience. There are people who prefer to say very little. Some come up with insights that none of the rest of us have thought of. People share experiences relating to the training and how it helped them, or come up with ideas for new things to try out. Most humbling of all is when people share deeply personal experiences, sometimes professional, sometimes just life experiences. The trust and bonds that develop in a good group goes beyond words.

I'll leave you with my personal thoughts on what Systema "is", or at least one way it can be viewed. Human beings consist of the following:

1. Nervous System
2. Cardiovascular System
3. Respiratory System
4. Genito-urinary System
5. Digestive System
6. Lymphatic/immune System
7. Muscular-skeletal System

In addition we might be said to possess physical, psychological and spiritual aspects to our make

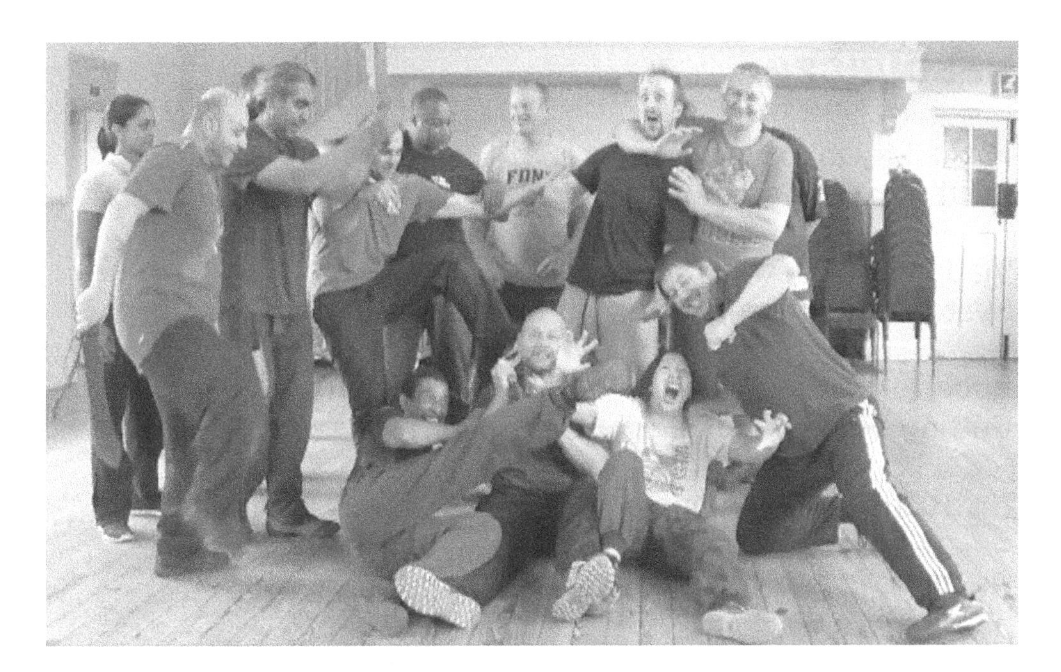

up. Training in Systema is designed to work on and through each and every one of these systems. Frequently an exercise might work on several systems at once. Even a simple push-up can be working on the respiratory, muscular and psychological systems simultaneously. Systema is designed to bring you personally an awareness of all of these systems and their strengths and weaknesses.

So one way to approach your work is to think what "systems" you would like to train and adapt your exercise accordingly. As Vladimir describes, this is also why Systema can be called *poznai sebia* or Know Yourself. This, on all sorts of levels, promotes our understanding of ourselves.

When we work with other people we have an even greater opportunity for learning. Other people can be helpful, difficult, stubborn, kind or cruel, just as we can ourselves. Each of these states gives as a chance to learn something more about ourselves and how we react in different circumstances. This is alongside all the obvious traits we develop from partner training, such as increased awareness, camaraderie and so on.

As I have written before, if you can truly understand yourself and others, then self defence, survival, in fact life in general, takes on a different perspective. Doing what is necessary in any situation becomes clearer. Understanding destroys the two biggest killers – fear (stress) and ego (pride). Good luck in your training!

RESOURCES

Mikhail Ryabko
Systema HQ Moscow www.systemaryabko.com

Vladimir Vasiliev
Systema HQ Toronto www.russianmartialart.com

Robert Poyton
Cutting Edge Systema www.systemauk.com

Instructional Downloads www.systemafilms.com

RECOMMENDED READING

Strikes - Vladimir Vasiliev & Scott Meredith

Let Every Breath - Vladimir Vasiliev

The Systema Manual - Major Konstantin Komarov

The Ten Points of Sparring - Robert Poyton

Systema Solo Training - Robert Poyton

Systema Health - Matt Hill

Systema Combat Drills - Matt Hill

NOTES